Documentation for Physical Therapist Assistants

Second Edition

Marianne Lukan, MA, BS, PT
Instructor
Physical Therapist Assistant Program
Lake Superior College
Duluth, Minnesota

F.A. Davis Company • Philadelphia

F. A. Davis Company

1915 Arch Street
Philadelphia, PA 19103
www.fadavis.com

Publisher: Jean François-Vilain
Developmental Editor: Sharon Lee
Production Editors: Bette Haitsch and Jack Brandt
Designer: Christine Cantera
Cover Designer: Louis J. Forgione

As new scientific information becomes available through basic and clinical research, recommended treatments and drug therapies undergo changes. The author(s) and publisher have done everything possible to make this book accurate, up to date, and in accord with accepted standards at the time of publication. The authors, editors, and publisher are not responsible for errors or omissions or for consequences from application of the book, and make no warranty, expressed or implied, in regard to the contents of the book. Any practice described in this book should be applied by the reader in accordance with professional standards of care used in regard to the unique circumstances that may apply in each situation. The reader is advised always to check product information (package inserts) for changes and new information regarding dose and contraindications before administering any drug. Caution is especially urged when using new or infrequently ordered drugs.

Library of Congress Cataloging in Publication Data

Lukan, Marianne, 1940—
    Documentation for physical therapist assistants / Marianne Lukan.—
2nd ed.
        p. cm.
    Includes bibliographical references and index.
    ISBN 0-8036-0837-3
    1. Physical therapy assistants.   2. Physical
therapy—Documentation.   3. Medical records.   I. Title.
    RM705 .L84 2001
    615.8'2—dc21

                                          2001028198

➤ PREFACE

The response from students and instructors alike to the first edition of *Documentation for Physical Therapist Assistants* was very gratifying. Before starting a revision, I decided to conduct a survey of instructors who used the first edition to get their recommendations for the second edition. While the responses to that survey were many and varied, the three most frequently requested changes were to: (1) make the text compatible with the *Guide to Physical Therapist Practice,* a reference published by the American Physical Therapy Association (APTA), providing guidelines for physical therapy patient/client management and scope of practice; (2) add more information to Chapter 7 ("Writing the Content: Diagnoses, Functional Outcomes, Goals, and Treatment Effectiveness"); and (3) add more practice exercises. I have tried to honor these requests as best I can in this, the second edition.

GUIDE TO PHYSICAL THERAPIST PRACTICE

The terminology and definitions used in the second edition are based on the terminology and definitions in the *Guide*. Evaluations are now referred to as examinations and evaluations. In Chapters 5 and 6 ("Writing the Content: Subjective Data" and "Writing the Content: Objective Data"), the reader is instructed to relate the progress note information to the physical therapist's initial examination. In Chapters 7 and 8, the reader is instructed to relate the progress note information to the physical therapist's initial evaluation. The title of Chapter 8 is "Writing the Content: Intervention Plan." The PTA performs and documents data collection skills and interventions, rather than assessing and applying modalities. Expected functional outcomes and anticipated goals replace long-term and short-term goals. Physical therapy diagnosis replaces physical therapy problem.

EXPANSION OF CHAPTER 7

Chapter 7 was expanded to include additional information on writing functional outcomes and goals. The chapter also features a discussion about how the PTA can make clinical decisions regarding the design and progression of each treatment session based on the information in the PT goals and intervention plan.

ADDITIONAL PRACTICE EXERCISES

Conscious of how much our students pay for textbooks, I feared that adding more practice exercises would increase both the book's physical size and its cost. My solution was to add an Instructor's Guide that would accompany the text and include most of the extra practice exercises. (Chapters 2 and 7 in the text also have new practice exercises.) The extra practice exercises in the Instructor's Guide can be used for homework assignments or tests. To allow for additional class activities and discussion, homework assignments, or tests, I removed the answers to some of the practice exercises from the text and placed them in the new Instructor's Guide.

ADDITIONAL REQUESTS

Several survey participants requested a section on writing for reimbursement. While I can understand their concern, I believe that we should be cautious about specifically "writing for reimbursement" because doing so places too much emphasis on wording. If the guidelines and theories in the text are followed, the documentation will be clear and will reflect quality patient care. If the documentation clearly describes the necessity for the skills of a trained physical therapy provider, there should be no problem with reimbursement.

For similar reasons, I also did not elaborate on Medicare documentation or computer documentation, as requested by a few instructors. Medicare documentation is subject to change and computer documentation is dependent on the individual software used. Again, if the guidelines in the text are followed, the documentation can be adapted to Medicare and computer formats.

—Marianne Lukan

➤ ACKNOWLEDGMENTS

I want to thank everyone who responded to the survey and commend PTA educators who are so willing to share information and ideas. I have recognized those who contributed suggestions for the Instructor's Guide in its introduction. I am grateful to Stephanie Lunning, former Peer Review Director of the Minnesota Chapter of the American Physical Therapy Association, for providing advice from the perspective of the third party payer, and to Barbara Struck, instructor for the medical transcriptionist program at Lake Superior College, for her input. I also want to thank Sharon Lee and Maryann Foley, development editors at F.A. Davis, and Marcia Craig, senior production editor at Graphic World Publishing Services, for their expertise and help in the revisions and the incorporation of the APTA terminology from the *Guide to Physical Therapist Practice* and APTA Documentation Guidelines.

➤ CONTENTS

PART ONE

Why Document?

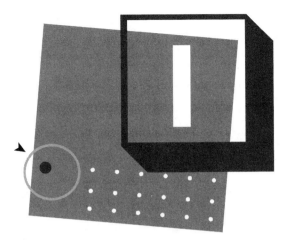

Introduction to Documentation

LEARNING OBJECTIVES

After studying this chapter, the student will be able to:
➤ Define documentation
➤ Describe changes in referral for physical therapy that have occurred since the early 1960s.
➤ Explain how changes in referral for physical therapy affected the evolution of responsibilities for the PT and PTA
➤ Identify the major factor that currently influences provision of health-care services and PT/PTA responsibilities
➤ Describe the role of documentation in patient care
➤ Discuss how documentation benefits the PTA, patient, and PT profession

INTRODUCTION

As an educator, I frequently hear students tell me they chose to become physical therapist assistants (PTAs), working with patients daily, because they had heard that physical therapists (PTs) spend all their time doing evaluations and completing paperwork. However, thorough and proper documentation is the responsibility of both the PT and the PTA. This book discusses the documentation tasks expected from the PTA, the importance of quality documentation, and the best way to produce thorough and proper documentation.

DOCUMENTATION AND ITS SIGNIFICANCE

Webster's dictionary defines *document* as "anything written that gives information or supplies evidence." *Documentation* is defined as "the assembling of documents, the using of documentary evidence to support original written work, or the evidence itself . . . , the classifying and making available of knowledge as a procedure."[1]

Evidence of Patient Care

In any health-care facility, services are provided to the patient by more than one caregiver. Records or medical charts are kept to document treatments, services performed, and services to be provided. Medical charts provide information that authenticates care given to the patient and reasons for providing that care. Thus, documentation is written proof that medical care was given to the patient, and this evidence is available for future use. If the treatment provided is not documented in the chart, it is assumed the treatment was not provided. "If it isn't written, it didn't happen" is a good rule.

Accountability for Patient Care

The written record is the mechanism through which the caregiver is held accountable for the medical care provided. The record is reviewed by the third-party payer to determine the reimbursement value of the medical services, and the information is studied to measure or determine the efficacy of the treatment procedures. The reader of the medical record finds the rationale that supports the medical necessity of the treatment.

Importance of Documentation

The impact of poorly written physical therapy documentation is illustrated in the following story based on a true experience of mine in 1968. The situation includes some of the topics and information discussed in this text. However, in some particulars, the situation only alludes to this information. A practice exercise after the last chapter challenges the reader to identify these topics.

The Experience

The telephone ring startled the baby and interrupted the relaxed after-dinner mood in the kitchen. My husband and I were chatting about the day, my busy patient schedule at the local hospital, and his insurance sales while our 3-month-old baby napped.

Answering the phone, I immediately heard, "I finally found you! You are to be in court in The City 3 days from now to testify for my client, Tony T. Do you remember him? I will meet with you in my office the night before to go over the medical records and your physical therapy notes."

My stomach did a flip-flop and my heart raced! I certainly did remember Tony. I was his physical therapist 5 years earlier when I lived in The City. I did not remember all the details of his treatments, and the thought of testifying at a jury trial struck terror in my heart! The lawyer assured me that he had my progress notes, and I would have time to review them before I was called to testify.

Settled in the lawyer's office, I looked over Tony's medical chart, which contained a record of his medical care when he was in the hospital and when he came to the physical therapy department as an outpatient. I reviewed the notes I had written about his physical therapy evaluations and treatment (Fig. 1–1). This documentation was in my familiar, illegible handwriting. My notes were only two to three lines in length, and as I read them, they actually told me nothing. Instead of my signature, I saw just the initials of my name when I was single. I marveled at how the lawyer started with those initials and proceeded to find me, now married and living in another part of the state!

Tony had dived into a shallow pool, hitting his head on the bottom and fracturing a vertebra in his neck. Although this caused some damage to his spinal cord, it was not completely severed. Tony had quadriparesis, weakness of varying degrees in his arms, legs, and trunk. His condition gradually improved, and his therapy consisted of exercises and activities to improve the strength, coordination, and endurance needed for him to become independent in all his functional activities. Left with disability, he was suing the owners of the pool. The opposition was fighting to keep the settlement low. They thought there was evidence that he could have been more cooperative and conscientious with his physical therapy.

My documentation followed the format commonly used by therapists in the hospital at that time. These progress notes certainly wouldn't meet the present criteria for third-party payers such as Medicare! How was I going to respond to cross-examination by the opposing lawyer, when my notes simply said "pt. improving" and "pt. tolerated treatment well"? They didn't help me recall the specifics of Tony's physical therapy treatments that I needed to tes-

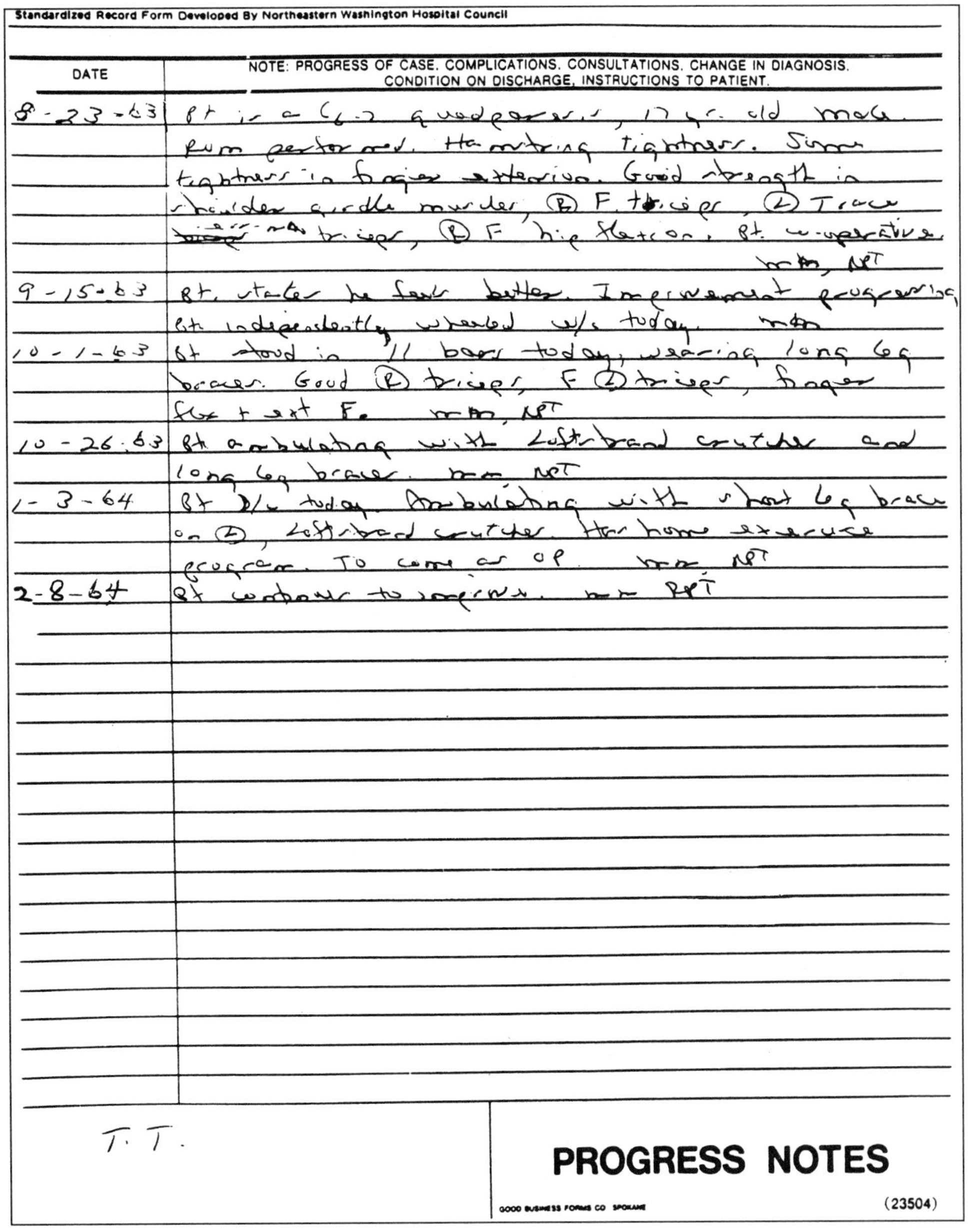

Figure 1–1 A page from the medical chart containing the physical therapy progress notes for Tony T. written before 1968.

tify. How I wished these notes had been better written! Somehow, we deciphered the notes, I recalled the information, and I was ready to testify.

During the trip home, my thoughts were consumed by the importance of quality documentation. My court experience would have been so much easier if I had written my notes then in the same format as I do now. What a difference! (Definitions of the abbreviations used in the following note are in Appendix A.)

2-8-64: Pt. has attended outpatient physical therapy 10× since hospital d/c, no-show for appts 1-16, 23, 25, and 2-6-64.

S: Pt. c/o his legs feel "tighter" than usual, states he stopped doing his home exercises because "they're boring, would rather play chess." He doesn't know why he did not come to all his therapy appointments.

O: Pt. ambulates ① using R forearm crutch & L AFO. He demonstrates occasional loss of balance but able to ① regain balance & does not fall. He circumducts his L leg during initial and mid-swing with inadequate hip and knee flexion. Hypertonus in hip extensor & quadriceps muscles palpable. Active SLR 0–50° bilaterally, 0–30° last week. Pt. uses 5-lb cuff wt. for 30 reps active knee flexion bilaterally, in prone position, up 1 lb from last week. Following 15 sec of pelvic rotation and wt.-shifting movements, pt. able to use hip & knee flexion during gait to step over cuff wts lying on the floor. Pt. instructed to always do a few rotational and wt.-shifting movements just before walking to ↓ mm tone. Pt. ambulated c̄ straight cane, min. assist for balance control, 100 ft on tiled, level surface. Pt. correctly demonstrated home ex. program modified to include walking while wearing cuff wts, beginning with 2 lb, & doing concentric and eccentric ex. on stairs. Please refer to written instructions in chart.

MMT finger flexion/extension	2-8-64	1-3-64
right	F	F
left	P	P

Exercises include using his lightest chess pieces, then progressing to his heavier pieces to strengthen finger flexion.

A: Improvement in pt.'s hamstring strength and ability to control extensor hypertonus to improve quality of gait. Potential for meeting goal of ① community ambulation c̄ straight cane is good. Finger strength status quo, possibly a result of not exercising. Exercises changed to be more interesting and motivating for pt.

P: Pt. scheduled 2×/week for 2 weeks to monitor home exercise program & ambulation progress. Will focus on ambulation c̄ cane on stairs, carpet, and grass next session.

—Marianne Mouser, PT Lic. #123

EVOLUTION OF PT/PTA RESPONSIBILITIES AND THE ROLE OF DOCUMENTATION

This 1968 event is an example of how documentation has evolved over time. This change has been a result of the changing responsibilities of the PT and the PTA.

The Past

Two events have influenced the evolution of PT and PTA treatment and documentation responsibilities and the role of documentation in patient care. These two events are changes in physician referral for physical therapy and the enactment of Medicare insurance.

Changes in Physician Referrral for Physical Therapy

The method by which physicians prescribe physical therapy has changed throughout the profession's short history. The changes have increased the PT's clinical decision-making power, led to the development of the physical therapy diagnosis, and offered the opportunity for autonomy.

THE PHYSICAL THERAPY PRESCRIPTION. Until the early 1960s, patients commonly came to a PT with referrals from physicians in the form of physical therapy prescriptions. That is, they read much like a medication prescription, as illustrated in Figure 1–2, or the instructions were more general, such as ultrasound, massage, or exercise. The PT was required to follow the physician's orders and provide the treatment as prescribed. If the PT did not agree with the treatment plan, he or she needed to discuss this with the physician in an attempt to agree on a more appropriate treatment plan. The PT was not always successful in convincing the physician to change the order; thus, the physical therapy treatment provided may not have been as effective as possible. The PT was practicing at the level of a technician, following precise directions from the physician and documenting briefly that the treatment was provided and whether the patient was improving.

EVALUATE AND TREAT. In the early 1960s, PTs began convincing some physicians that PTs had the training and knowledge to evaluate a patient's neuromusculoskeletal system and de-

---

P. T. Knowes, MD
123 Medical Building
Yourtown, AZ 12345
(001) 222-3333

Physical Therapy for Hazel Jones

US at 1.5 w/cm^2 for 5 min to the right deltoid insertion, followed by 10 min of massage.
AAROM 10 reps for abduction, flexion, and external rotation.

P.T. Knowes, MD

Figure 1–2 Illustration of a physician's order for physical therapy that tells the physical therapist exactly what to do. It resembles a medication prescription.

termine the treatment appropriate for the patient's condition. Patients brought referrals from their physicians that provided the diagnosis and stated "evaluate and treat." The responsibility of the PT expanded to include (1) determining the physical therapy diagnosis based on results of the evaluation; and (2) defining the interventions or treatment plan. The physical therapy problem would be described in terms of the neuromusculoskeletal abnormality, and the treatment plan would be directed toward correcting or minimizing this problem. The PT needed evaluation skills to identify physical therapy problems and to make clinical decisions regarding treatment of those problems. Writing the initial, interim, and discharge evaluations became additional documentation responsibilities.

The first academic program for training the PTA was established in 1967. The PTA became the technician providing the physical therapy treatments under the direct guidance and supervision of the PT. Writing progress notes was a documentation responsibility shared by the PT and PTA.

DIRECT ACCESS. Direct access allows a person access to the medical care system directly through a PT. The PT may evaluate the patient to determine whether the patient's condition is a disorder treatable by physical therapy without a physician's referral. Nebraska has allowed direct access since 1957. California eliminated the need for a physician's referral in 1968. When Maryland's Physical Therapy Practice Act was amended in 1979 to allow direct access, many American Physical Therapy Association (APTA) state chapters launched their amendment campaigns. Today, the only five states that do not have direct-access language in their state practice acts[2] have direct-access legislation in progress.

Direct access gives the PT opportunity for autonomy, but it also requires the PT to have the skills and knowledge to recognize conditions that are not problems that can be helped by physical therapy. The PT is responsible for referring a patient to a physician or other appropriate health-care provider if the patient exhibits signs and symptoms of a systemic disorder or a problem that is beyond the scope or expertise of the PT. The PTA is responsible for reporting any signs or symptoms or lack of progress that indicates a need for PT reevaluation or referral to a physician or other health-care provider.

The focus of PT education has had to change, increasing the emphasis on scientific knowledge, evaluation skills, and critical thinking and research and decreasing the emphasis on treatment skills. PTA training, although still focusing on treatment skills, has expanded to emphasize the theories behind these treatment skills. This expansion provides the PTA with the knowledge to make clinical decisions within the parameters of the PT treatment plan and PTA level of training. In some areas, PTA responsibilities have evolved to allow PTAs to treat patients when the PT is not on the premises but is accessible by telephone.

Establishment of Medicare

Before 1970, documentation in the medical chart was not always thorough or specific. Health-care providers knew documentation should be done well, but unfortunately poor-quality documentation was easy to find. Typically, progress notes were brief, consisting of one or two lines, and subjective and/or judgmental in nature. For example: "Patient feeling better today" (see Fig. 1–1). No standards for documentation existed, and those paying the health-care bills did not demand accountability for those bills.

In the mid-1960s, this changed when the Health Insurance for the Aged and Disabled Act, known as Medicare, was enacted. Thus, the federal government was purchasing medical care for the elderly. Within the Department of Health and Human Services, the Health Care Financing Administration issued standards for documentation to be followed with all patients receiving Medicare. Other insurance companies soon followed Medicare's example. Those paying the medical bills demanded that health-care providers be held accountable for the dollars spent. This accountability was determined through proper documentation that clearly identified the physical therapy problem, treatment goals and plans, and treatment results.

The Present   Our health-care system is now in a state of transition; services provided to patients are being curtailed because of limited financial resources. The physical therapy provider is placed in a position of competing for these limited funds. Physical therapy services will not be reimbursed if the treatments are not effective and efficient. The patient or client seeks physical therapy because problems resulting from a disease or injury prevent the person from functioning in his or her environment. Interventions are directed toward improving or restoring the patient's functional abilities by minimizing or resolving the problems in the most cost-effective manner. Documentation that meets today's standards provides the basis for research to measure functional outcomes and identify the most effective and efficient treatment procedures. Documentation must describe what functional activities the patient has difficulty performing and show how the interventions are effective in improving or restoring the patient's function. Documentation must be done properly if PTs and PTAs are to survive financially.

ROLE OF DOCUMENTATION IN PATIENT CARE   Three themes are repeated in this text: (1) documentation records the quality of patient care; (2) documentation constructs a legal report of patient care; and (3) documentation provides the basis for reimbursement for patient care.

A Record of the Quality of Patient Care   The term *quality care* as used in this text refers to medical care that is appropriate for and focused on the patient's problems relevant to the diagnosis. *Quality physical therapy care* is defined as care that follows the *Standards of Practice* for physical therapy published by the American Physical Therapy Association (APTA).[3]

To provide high-quality medical care, good communication among caregivers is absolutely essential. The PTA must communicate with the PT. The PTA may also share and coordinate information with other providers of medical services, such as other PTs and PTAs who may fill in when the PTA is absent, occupational therapists and occupational therapy assistants, nurses and nursing assistants, physicians and physician assistants, speech pathologists, psychologists, social workers, and chaplains. The medical record is the avenue through which the medical team communicates regarding:

1. Identification of the patient's problems
2. Solutions
3. Plans for the patient's discharge
4. Coordination of the continuum of care

This communication process helps ensure the quality of care.

The quality of care provided by the medical facility is determined by a review of the existing records. This review process is a way to monitor and influence the quality of health care provided by the facility. The information in the medical record is reviewed or audited for three purposes: (1) quality assurance; (2) research and education; and (3) reimbursement.

1. Records are reviewed to determine whether the health care provided meets standards and criteria. This is done externally by agencies accrediting the facility and internally by a quality-assurance committee. Problem areas are identified and plans are made for correction and improvement. This is a continuous process; the quality assurance committee usually meets monthly, and agencies accredit facilities every 5 to 10 years. PTAs are permitted to serve on the quality-assurance committee.

2. Information in the medical record is used for research and student instruction. Research helps validate treatment techniques and identify new and better ways to provide health care. The record is used for retrospective studies that measure outcomes to determine the most cost-effective treatment approach to patient care. Students are encouraged to question and challenge treatment procedures as part of their learning process.

3. Third-party payers such as insurance companies and Medicare decide how to reimburse for medical care by reading the documentation in the medical record. The record must show that the patient's problems were identified and treatment was directed toward solving those problems and discharging the patient.

Documentation Standards and Criteria

Documentation that ensures quality care follows the standards and criteria set by a variety of sources. Although the standards are similar, the PTA should be familiar with the criteria required by:

1. The federal government
2. The state government
3. Professional agencies
4. Accrediting agencies
5. The health-care facility

FEDERAL GOVERNMENT. The federal government funds and administers Medicare. The PTA must follow Medicare documentation requirements when treating a patient with this type of insurance. Because these requirements change frequently and can become complicated, the PTA must stay informed and up-to-date in his or her knowledge of Medicare requirements.

STATE GOVERNMENT. Although funded by the federal government, Medicaid, a government program providing health care to the poor, is administered by the individual state governments. The state government funds medical assistance and workers' compensation requiring specific documentation criteria for patients with these types of insurance. The state may ask that specific data from the medical record be reported annually. Other documentation criteria determined at the state level may be influenced by the state's physical therapy legislation. The PTA must be well informed about his or her state's Physical Therapy Practice Act.

PROFESSIONAL AGENCIES. Professional agencies recommend documentation standards, such as the APTA's *Guidelines for Physical Therapy Documentation.*[4] These standards are the basis for the documentation instructions in this text and can be found in Appendix F.

ACCREDITING AGENCIES. Accrediting agencies provide standards that health-care facilities must follow to meet accreditation criteria, including documentation requirements. Hospitals are accredited by the Joint Commission on Accreditation of Healthcare Organizations. Rehabilitation facilities are accredited by the Commission on Accreditation of Rehabilitation Facilities.

HEALTH-CARE FACILITY. Each health-care facility has its own documentation criteria; most facilities incorporate federal, state, and professional standards into their own procedures. The PTA can follow all standards and criteria by remembering this good rule: Follow the policies and procedures of the facility where you work.

A Legal Record

The medical record and all that is contained within it comprise a legal document and legal proof of the quality of care provided. The record protects the patient and caregivers should any questions arise in the future regarding the patient's care.

Health-care providers work under the constant shadow of a possible malpractice lawsuit for each patient situation. Patients do become dissatisfied, often leading to questions about the care provided months or years after the patient received treatment. Often these questions result in lawsuits, and many cases go to court because of the patient's claim that injury or illness was caused by an accident or negligence on the part of someone else. PTs, and possibly PTAs, may be called on to testify in court. If the PT or PTA is called to testify, clear and accurate documentation is the best defense, demonstrating that safe and thorough patient care was provided.

A Basis for Reimbursement

The insurance company or organization paying for medical services determines the reimbursement rate from the information recorded in the medical chart. Payment is often denied when the documentation does not clearly provide the rationale to support the medical care that was provided. With some insurance plans, the caregiver must provide effective patient care while also containing the costs within a preset payment amount. The caregiver demonstrates accountability for these costs by thoroughly and properly documenting the care provided.

SUMMARY

Documenting in the medical record is one of the many responsibilities of the PTA. The medical record is a legal document that proves that medical care was given and holds the healthcare providers accountable for the quality of the care given. It is an avenue for constant communication among caregivers so goals can be identified and the treatment progress monitored. Insurance representatives read the medical record to determine whether to reimburse for the medical services provided.

Historically, PTs were technicians, providing physical therapy treatments that were prescribed in detail by the physician. Responsibilities have evolved such that PTs are now evaluators, consultants, managers, and practitioners seeing patients (clients) without a physician's referral. PTAs provide treatment under the guidance and supervision of the PT.

Physical therapy services must be provided in an efficient and cost-effective manner because financial resources to fund health care are no longer readily available. The outcomes now must focus on improving the client's functional abilities. Research must be done to measure outcomes or results of physical therapy procedures and define the most effective and efficient treatments to accomplish the functional goals. Proper documentation facilitates this research.

The provision of up-to-date and valid physical therapy services will be ensured through documentation that follows standards and criteria determined by federal and state governments, professional agencies, accrediting agencies, and the individual clinical facility. Although documentation formats differ from facility to facility, all incorporate the professional standards and criteria. The PTA should follow the policies and procedures of his or her clinical facility. Documenting according to standards and legal guidelines will produce a medical record that protects the patient and the PTA if the medical record is used in court proceedings.

REFERENCES

1. Cayne, BS (ed): The New Lexicon Webster's Dictionary of the English Language. Lexicon Publications, New York, 1989, p 276.2.
2. American Physical Therapy Association. Direct access to physical therapy services. States that permit physical therapy treatment without referral. http://www.apta.org/Advocacy/state/directaccess/State3 (accessed 9/4/00).
3. American Physical Therapy Association: Standards of Practice. APTA, Alexandria, VA, June 1999.
4. American Physical Therapy Association: Guidelines for Physical Therapy Documentation. APTA, Alexandria, VA, November 1998.

➤ Review Exercises

1. Describe what is meant by the following rule: "If it isn't written, it didn't happen."

2. Describe the changes in referral for physical therapy that have occurred since the early 1960s.

3. Discuss how changes in referral for physical therapy influenced the evolution of the responsibilities of the PT and the PTA.

4. Define *direct access.*

5. Identify the major factor currently influencing the provision of health-care services and PT/PTA responsibilities.

6. Describe three purposes for the medical record.

7. Explain why the medical record is audited.

8. Identify who determines standards or criteria for documentation.

9. Explain why the PTA should use the rule "follow the policies and procedures at the facility where you work."

Documentation Content

LEARNING OBJECTIVES

After studying this chapter, the student will be able to:
- ➤ Identify the six categories of documentation content
- ➤ Briefly describe the content to be documented in each category
- ➤ Differentiate PT and PTA documentation responsibilities
- ➤ Identify the five elements of physical therapy patient management
- ➤ Discuss the PTA's involvement with the different types of physical therapy evaluations

INTRODUCTION

The medical record is the written account of a patient's medical care. The content describes the medical care provided from the patient's admission through discharge.

Documentation content can be grouped into six categories:

1. Data relevant to the patient's condition
2. The problem(s) requiring medical treatment
3. Treatment plan or action to address the problem(s)
4. Goals or outcomes of the treatment plan
5. Record of administration of the treatment plan
6. Treatment effectiveness or results of the treatment plan

This information is found in the written evaluations, progress notes, and specialized test results such as radiography department and laboratory reports. Each content area is briefly described to provide an overview of the content of the medical record. In-depth explorations of these content areas for physical therapy documentation are discussed in Chapters 5 through 8.

DATA   Information gathered about a patient may include both subjective and objective data. Most of this information is gathered at the time of admission or the first time the patient is seen by each medical service provider. However, information is being gathered continuously throughout the span of the patient's care. Data gathered when the patient is admitted will be located in the reports of the initial examinations performed by the various medical services. For example, a young male student is admitted to the emergency department (ED) at XXX hospital at 2:45 AM Saturday after being involved in a motorcycle accident. Information is gathered at admission to the ED, when the patient is taken to radiography, when the patient is admitted to the orthopedic hospital unit, and when laboratory tests are performed. More information will be gathered when the patient is first seen by physical therapy, occupational therapy, and social services. Examples of the data gathered by each discipline are highlighted in Table 2–1.

Subjective Data   Information told to the health-care provider comprises subjective data. Subjective data include:

1. Information about the patient's past medical history
2. Symptoms or complaints that caused the patient to seek medical attention
3. Factors that produced the symptoms
4. The patient's functional and lifestyle needs
5. The patient's goals or expectations from medical care

Table 2–1 ➤ EXAMPLES OF DATA GATHERED BY VARIOUS SERVICES FOR A PATIENT IN A MOTORCYCLE ACCIDENT

Discipline/Service	Data
Admitting clerk	Past admission to the hospital Insurance information Nearest relative General information about the accident
Physician	Past medical history Detailed information about the accident Physical examination Orthopedic examination results from orthopedic surgeon Diagnostic and laboratory test results, such as x-rays
Nurse	Vital signs Bowel and bladder function Skin condition General nutritional status General ability for self-care, communication, and decision making
Physical therapist	Flexibility or joint range of motion Muscle strength Sensation Posture Ability to move about in environment
Occupational therapist	Specific ability for self-care in activities of daily living Vocational abilities Homemaking abilities General vision, hearing, and communication abilities
Social worker	Home environment and lifestyle More specific financial concerns General emotional development Family support and family adjustment

Typically, data relevant to the patient's condition and reason for admission are obtained by interviewing the patient or significant others.

Collecting subjective data is an ongoing process while medical care is being provided. The information reflects the patient's response to treatment and the effectiveness of treatment. The PT and PTA seek information provided by the patient . The PT documents subjective data in the physical therapy examination reports. The PTA documents subjective data in the daily or weekly progress notes.

Objective Data

Objective information includes information that is reproducible and readily demonstrable, gathered by carefully examining the patient using data-collecting methods such as measurements, tests, and observations. These methods can be reproduced by any medical professional with the same training as the one who first performed the examination.

Objective data are the signs of the patient's condition. Reviewing the signs by repeating the measurements, tests, and observations is also an ongoing process for determining treatment effectiveness and patient progress. The PT performs the physical therapy examination/evaluation and uses objective methods to gather data. These data are used to determine the physical therapy diagnosis. The PTA repeats any measurements, tests, and observations within the scope of his or her PTA training to determine the patient's progress toward accomplishing the treatment goals.

THE PROBLEM REQUIRING MEDICAL TREATMENT

The medical team identifies the patient's medical problems based on the data collected by the various disciplines. The physician determines the medical diagnosis, and other professionals identify problems that are treatable within their respective disciplines. The diagnosis is documented by the physician in the medical chart, usually near the beginning of the chart in a section specified for the physician's report. The identification of the physical therapy problem, called the *physical therapy diagnosis,* is usually documented in the physical therapy initial evaluation, located in either the physical therapy section or the evaluation section of the chart. Other problems are discussed in other health-care providers' evaluations. Possible problems identified by the physicians, nurses, and social worker examining the student in the motorcycle accident example may include the following:

1. Compound fracture of the shaft of right femur
2. Lacerations into quadriceps muscles
3. Infected open wound
4. Edema of the right foot
5. Questionable chemical dependency
6. Fever
7. Elevated blood pressure

Definition of Terms

Some terms need to be defined before comparing the medical diagnoses with the physical therapy diagnosis. The preferred practice patterns of physical therapy outlined by The American Physical Therapy Association (APTA) in the *Guide to Physical Therapist Practice** are based on a process of disablement. This process describes a chain of events beginning with a pathology, which may lead to impairments, which may lead to functional limitations, which may lead to a disability. *Impairment* is defined as "loss or abnormality of physiological, psychological, or anatomical structure or function."[1] *Functional limitation* is "restriction of the ability to perform—at the level of the whole person—a physical action, activity, or task in an efficient, typically expected, or competent manner."[1] *Disability* refers to "the inability to engage in age-specific, gender-specific, or sex-specific roles in a particular social context and physical environment."[1]

---

*The *Guide to Physical Therapist Practice* is a publication by The American Physical Therapy Association that describes the following: (1) physical therapists and their roles in health care; (2) the generally accepted elements of physical therapy patient/client management; (3) types of tests and measurements used by physical therapists; (4) types of interventions physical therapists use; (5) the anticipated goals of the interventions; and (6) the expected outcomes of physical therapy patient/client management. Preferred practice patterns are descriptions about common physical therapy management strategies for specific diagnostic groups. The patterns serve as a guide for the physical therapist when planning comprehensive plans of care.

This disablement framework is a variation of the model describing the implication of pathology issued by the World Health Organization (WHO). The terminology in this model, the International Classification of Impairments, Disabilities, and Handicaps (ICIDH), is used in the international physical therapy community. The ICIDH term *disability* is equivalent to APTA's *functional limitation,* and the ICIDH term *handicap* has the same meaning as APTA's *disability.* It should be noted that at the time of this writing, WHO is in the process of changing this terminology. The new proposal is ICIDH-2: *International Classification of Functioning and Disability.* "'Functioning' and 'disability' are umbrella terms covering three dimensions: (1) body functions and structure; (2) activities at the individual level; and (3) participation in society."[2] This new terminology is in line with APTA's impairments, functional limitation, and disability terms. Final adoption of these new terms is expected sometime in 2001.[2]

Medical Diagnosis

The medical diagnosis is of a systemic disease or disorder, which is determined by the physician's evaluation and diagnostic tests. "Diagnosis is the recognition of disease. It is the determination of the cause and nature of pathologic conditions."[3] The medical diagnosis is equivalent to the pathology in the APTA and ICIDH models. In the example of the student in the motorcycle accident, the medical diagnosis was "a fractured femur and infected lacerations."

Physical Therapy Problem: Diagnosis

The physical therapy problem is not a medical diagnosis. According to Sahrmann,[4] the physical therapy problem is the identification of pathokinesiologic (i.e., study of movements related to a given disorder) problems associated with faulty biomechanical or neuromuscular action.[4] In Sahrmann's definition, faulty biomechanical or neuromuscular action is now termed *impairments,* and pathokinesiologic problems are now called *functional limitations.* In the APTA model, the physical therapy diagnosis consists of the patient's impairments and functional limitations, whereas in the ICIDH model the physical therapy diagnosis consists of the patient's impairments and disabilities. In both models, the physical therapy treatment objectives are aimed at eliminating or minimizing the impairments and functional limitations or disabilities. The desired outcome of the physical therapy treatment is preventing or minimizing the severity of the disability or handicap.

Impairments

Impairments are abnormalities or dysfunctions of the bones, joints, ligaments, muscles, tendons, nerves, and skin, or problems with movement resulting from a pathology in the brain, spinal cord, pulmonary, or cardiovascular systems. A few common examples of dysfunctions treatable by PT include muscle weakness; tendon inflammation; connective tissue tightness with limited range of motion (ROM) in the joints; muscle spasms; edema; and difficulties moving in bed, moving from sitting to standing, and walking. Impairments in the physical therapy diagnosis may be the same as in the medical diagnosis (e.g., "a rotated L5 vertebra," with muscle spasms and pain limiting a truck driver's sitting tolerance to 5 minutes). The physician, after determining that the L5 vertebra is rotated on the basis of x-rays and examination, may indicate this as the medical diagnosis. If the patient went to see the PT first, the PT, after performing the examination, may identify the rotated vertebra. This, plus the muscle spasms, is the musculoskeletal dysfunction part of the physical therapy diagnosis. A patient may have a medical diagnosis with a physical therapy diagnosis (e.g., rheumatoid arthritis with adhesive capsulitis of the anterior capsule limiting shoulder ROM interfering with a retiree's ability to put on shirt and sweater). In the latter case, rheumatoid arthritis is the medical diagnosis, and adhesive capsulitis limiting shoulder ROM is part of the physical therapy diagnosis.

Functional Limitations

The definition of the physical therapy diagnosis must include the patient's functional abilities or inabilities. The patient comes to physical therapy because of an inability to function adequately in his or her environment. Using the previously cited examples, the student with the fractured femur will not be able to ambulate bearing weight on the fractured leg, the truck driver with the rotated L5 vertebra cannot sit longer than 5 minutes, and the retiree with rheumatoid arthritis cannot put on his shirt and sweater. These functional problems become the basis for determining the outcomes toward which the physical therapy treatments are directed, and the rate of progress toward accomplishing the goals and outcomes determines the duration of the physical therapy services.

Differentiating Between the Medical Diagnosis and Physical Therapy Diagnosis

The PTA should distinguish between the medical diagnosis and the physical therapy diagnosis when treating and documenting. Examples of medical diagnoses include the following:

1. Multiple sclerosis
2. Rheumatoid arthritis
3. Fractured right femur
4. Cerebral vascular accident secondary to thrombosis
5. Compression fracture of T12 vertebra with compression of spinal cord

Physical therapy diagnoses that may be associated with the medical diagnoses listed above are discussed in the following examples.

Diagnosis: Ataxia of lower extremities with inability to ambulate independently.

Discussion: A patient with the medical diagnosis of multiple sclerosis may have the physical therapy diagnosis of ataxia (the impairment) and the functional problem of inability to ambulate (the functional limitation). In the past, the result of the treatment was documented by a description of the improvement in impairment (e.g., pt.'s coordination improved as pt. able to place R heel on L knee). Today, treatment effectiveness is documented by a description of a decrease in the functional limitation, such as improvement in the ability or quality of the patient's ambulation (e.g., pt. able to walk to mailbox without assistive device but needs standby assist because of occasional loss of balance).

Diagnosis: ROM deficits in right shoulder limiting the ability to put on shirt and sweater.

Discussion: The patient with the medical diagnosis of rheumatoid arthritis may have the physical therapy diagnosis consisting of the impairment, ROM deficits, and the functional limitation (APTA) or disability (ICIDH) of difficulty in dressing. In the past, it was acceptable to document treatment effectiveness in degrees of increased ROM (e.g., shoulder flexion 0–100°, an improvement of 20° since initial eval.). Today, a description of the patient's ability to put on his or her shirt or sweater, along with the improvement in degrees of ROM, documents the treatment effectiveness (e.g., client able to put on loose-fitting pullover sweater without assistance) and puts meaning to the ROM degrees.

TREATMENT PLAN OR ACTION

The list of the patient's medical problems is used to plan the patient's medical treatment. Appropriate strategies for resolving or minimizing the problems are outlined by the various disciplines involved. These strategies are the treatment plans. In the case of the motorcycle accident patient, the physician would design a treatment plan for medication to stop the infection, and then for surgery to pin and stabilize the fractured femur. Nursing may design a treatment plan for positioning the right foot to reduce the edema and for monitoring blood pressure. The social worker may design a treatment plan to help the patient address his questionable chemical dependency. Later, the PT may design a treatment plan to teach the patient to walk with crutches. In the example of the truck driver, the PT may design a treatment plan to include applying a physical agent to relax muscle spasms, performing mobilization techniques to de-rotate the L5 vertebra, and educating the driver about sitting support and posture. These treatment plans, described in the medical record, include frequency and duration of the treatment procedures.

Informed Consent to the Treatment Plan

All aspects of the treatment plan, including the purposes, procedures, expected results, and any possible risks or side effects of treatment, must be explained to the patient and significant others. In some cases, the patient may participate in designing the plan. The patient or a representative for the patient should agree to the treatment plan and procedures. His or her decision to consent to the treatment (informed consent) is based on the information provided about the treatment. In many medical facilities, a formal informed consent form or document must be signed before treatment is initiated. When a patient is receiving physical therapy, the PT designs the treatment plan and reviews the plan with the patient. Thus, the appropriate person to obtain the informed consent signature is the PT, not the PTA. Once signed, this form is placed in the medical record.

GOALS AND OUTCOMES

All health-care providers identify the goals or outcomes to be accomplished by their treatment plans. In the case of the student involved in the motorcycle accident, the physician's goals may be to treat the infection and stabilize the fractured femur so healing can occur. The nurse's goals may be to monitor the patient and prevent any other problems as a result of the patient's injury and temporary inactivity. The social worker's goal may be to help the patient find the most appropriate resources and help for his chemical dependency.

The functional outcomes toward which the PT's treatment plan is directed should include the patient's expectations (i.e., what is meaningful to the patient) for eliminating or minimizing the patient's functional limitations. The physical therapy goals are directed at eliminating or minimizing the patient's impairments. Therefore, the physical therapy goals and outcomes are planned with patient and PT collaboration. The goals for the truck driver are to decrease his pain and improve his trunk ROM, whereas his functional outcome is to be able to sit for at least 2 hours so he can return to work. The student's functional outcome is to learn how to use crutches so he can return to college. The goals and outcomes give the PTA direction for planning the treatment sessions, progressing the treatment outlined in the PT's plan, and recommending the termination of treatment. The PT and the PTA need to stay focused on the purpose of the treatment plan, gearing everything done during a treatment session toward improving or resolving the functional problem that brought the client to physical therapy. Likewise, all documentation should be focused on the treatment appropriate for the goals and outcomes and on the progress toward accomplishing the functional outcomes.

RECORD OF ADMINISTRATION OF THE TREATMENT PLAN

The medical chart contains proof that the treatment plan is being carried out. Recording the administration of the treatment procedures can range from simply checking off items listed in a flow chart or checklist to writing a narration or report about the treatment in daily, weekly, or monthly progress notes.

Progress Note

The progress note is a recording of the treatment provided for each problem, the patient's reaction to the treatment procedures, progress toward goals and outcomes, and any changes in the patient's condition. Although both the PT and the PTA write the progress notes, this text is directed toward the skills needed by PTAs to write quality notes.

TREATMENT EFFECTIVENESS

This content area contains an interpretation of the patient's response to the treatment, the *most* important content in the medical record. It is considered the "bottom line" of the health-care business. Here, the caregiver documents whether or not goals were met, thus documenting the effectiveness of the treatment plan. This information tells the reader about the quality of the medical care provided. The researcher uses this content to measure outcomes and determine the efficacy of treatment procedures. The third-party payer reads this information to determine whether the medical care met the requirements for reimbursement.

THE EXAMINATION/ EVALUATION BY PHYSICAL THERAPY

Five Elements of Physical Therapy Patient Management

According to the *Guide to Physical Therapist Practice,* "the physical therapist integrates five elements of patient/client management—examination, evaluation, diagnosis, prognosis, and intervention—in a manner designed to maximize outcomes."[1] *Examination* is the process for gathering subjective and objective data about the patient. *Evaluation* is the clinical judgment the therapist makes based on the examination. The evaluation results in the determination of the diagnosis, prognosis, and interventions. The *prognosis* is a judgment about the level of optimal improvement the patient may attain and the amount of time needed to reach that level. *Interventions* are the skilled techniques and activities that make up the treatment plan.

Types and Content of Examination/ Evaluations

The PT should always perform an initial examination and evaluation and a discharge examination and evaluation of the patient, and may perform one or more interim evaluations, depending on the length of time the patient is receiving the physical therapy care. The PT follows the APTA *Guidelines for Physical Therapy Documentation*[5] outlining the recommended content of the reports. These Guidelines are in Appendix F in this text. A description of each type of examination/evaluation report follows this discussion with a list of the recommended information contained in the report. The medical record content categories discussed in this chapter are indicated in bold next to the physical therapy examination and evaluation information appropriate for each category to demonstrate how the physical therapy report conforms to the documentation content in the medical record.

Initial Examination/ Evaluation

This examination and evaluation are performed the first time the PT sees the patient. This written report contains the following information:

1. *History and risk factor identification.* General statistics about the patient are obtained before the evaluation is performed. Some of this information may be found elsewhere in the chart, such as in notes from admissions or the physician. Examples are age, medical diagnosis, name, sex, date of birth, physician, complications, and precautions. All of these data are required in the medical record but all may not be in the PT's evaluation if they are already located elsewhere in the chart.
2. **Subjective data:** Information is obtained from what the patient tells the PT or PTA during the interview. Examples are onset of injury/disease/pain, chief complaint, location of complaints, functional limitations, home situation, lifestyle, goals, and pertinent medical history.
3. Selecting and administering tests and measures: **Objective data:** Results of objective testing and observations. Examples are physical status, such as strength, endurance, skin condition, ROM, and neurologic status; functional status, such as mobility, transfers, ambulation, activities of daily living, and ability at work/school/home; and mental status, such as cognition, orientation, communication problems, judgment, and ability to follow directions.
4. Evaluation: PT's interpretation of the results of the testing and observations.
5. Diagnosis: The physical therapy **diagnosis** identifying the impairments and functional limitations.
6. Goals: Anticipated **goals and expected outcomes** related to resolving the diagnosis, written in measureable and functional terms.
7. Intervention plan or recommendation requirements: **Treatment plans** related to accomplishing the goals, including specific interventions, their frequency and duration, a statement regarding the prognosis (the patient's rehabilitation potential or expectations of treatment effectiveness), an estimate of the length of time the patient will be receiving physical therapy treatment, and a schedule or plan for evaluating the effectiveness of the treatment.
8. Authentication and appropriate designation of physical therapist, including signature, title, and professional license number.

Re-examination/ and Re-evaluation

Documentation of the continuum of physical therapy care that the patient is receiving is recorded by the PT in the re-examination and re-evaluation reports and by the PTA or PT in the progress notes. The content of the PT re-examination and re-evaluation is discussed below, and because it is the purpose of this book, the discussion of the content of the progress note is discussed in the remaining chapters.

Interim or progress examinations/evaluations are performed by the PT periodically throughout the period the patient is receiving physical therapy. The progress examination/ evaluation content includes the following:

1. Intervention or service provided: **Treatment procedures administered** involving a summary of the interventions and other services provided by the PT or PTA since the initial evaluation.
2. Patient status, progress, or regression: **Subjective data**—Patient's subjective information as to the effectiveness of the interventions. **Objective data**—A repeat of the testing and observations made in the initial examination.

3. Re-examination and re-evaluation: **Results or effectiveness of the treatment plan,** including:
   a. Interpretation of objective testing and observations and a comparison with the initial evaluation
   b. Statement addressing the accomplishment of goals set in the initial evaluation and any new goals set
   c. Information regarding any change in the patient's status
   d. Treatment plan written by the PT indicating whether the initial plan is to be continued or changed
   e. Signature, title, and license number of the physical therapist

Summation of Care   This discharge examination/evaluation is the patient's final evaluation and the final note about the patient in the medical record. This note must be written by the PT. A properly written discharge note follows the APTA guidelines and should include the following information:

1. Brief summary of the treatment that was provided (intervention procedures administered)
2. Relevant information provided by the patient (subjective data)
3. Interpretation of repeated testing and observations and a comparison with latest interim evaluation or initial evaluation (objective data and results or effectiveness of interventions)
4. Statement regarding accomplishment of anticipated goals and expected outcomes (results or effectiveness of the treatment plan)
5. Further interventions or care needed after discharge
6. Plans for follow-up or monitoring after discharge
7. Signature, title, and professional license number of the PT

DISCHARGE NOTES   Physical therapy professionals disagree about the definitions of *discharge evaluation* and *discharge summary.* Some believe the evaluation and the summary are the same, whereas others consider them different types of documents.

If a discharge summary is considered the same as a discharge evaluation, then the evaluation/summary will have content that interprets the testing results and identifies plans for the patient after discharge. Decisions about the patient's care after discharge may be made based on the information in the discharge evaluation/summary. In this case, only a PT can write a discharge summary.

When a patient's treatment has been discontinued, the PTA may write a discharge summary or note. This note only summarizes the care given the patient, summarizes the patient's response to the interventions, and states objectively the functional status of the patient at the time of discharge. No interpretation of the data or evaluation is made, no plan for the patient's care after discharge is identified, and no decisions are made based on the examination. If the physical therapy clinician writes discharge summaries of this nature, there still must be a discharge evaluation written by the PT as the final note in the patient's medical record. In any situation, the *final documentation in the patient's physical therapy chart must be written by the physical therapist.*

PTA Involvement   Although the PTA does not perform evaluations, he or she may assist the PT with the examination procedures. The PTA may take notes and help gather the subjective data. The PTA also may take measurements, perform some tests, and record the results. However, the PTA may not interpret the results. Performing the tests and recording the results constitute *data collection.* Interpreting the results involves making a judgment about their value. This is called *evaluating.* Examples of tests and measurements that are part of a PTA's data collection skills are girth measurements, manual muscle testing of muscle groups, goniometry measurements, and vital signs. During the course of a patient's treatment, the PTA often is expected to repeat the measurements and tests to record the patient's progress since the initial examination/evaluation. These objective data are more reliable when the same person performs the tests and measurements in a consistent manner throughout the course of the patient's treatment. In addition, assisting the PT with the examination offers the PTA and patient an opportunity to become acquainted so the patient will feel comfortable working with the PTA as the treatment plan is carried out.

When writing progress notes, the PTA refers to the problems, goals and outcomes, and treatment plans in the initial and interim evaluation reports. Progress notes should record the effectiveness of the treatment plan by comparing the patient's progress toward accomplishing the goals and outcomes with the status of the patient at initial evaluation.

Documentation Responsibilities

The documentation content is found in the examination/evaluation reports and progress notes. The PT is responsible for the evaluations, consultations, and decision making required for the patient's physical therapy health care. Therefore, the PT's documentation responsibilities are to record the:

1. Initial evaluation, which includes goals and outcomes and treatment plan
2. Interim or progress evaluations performed
3. Discharge information
4. Changes in the treatment plan

The PT may also write progress notes. The primary documentation responsibility of the PTA is to record the progress or interim notes.

The PTA must be familiar with the content of the PT examination/evaluation reports. The report informs the PTA of the patient's medical and physical therapy diagnoses. The PTA follows the treatment plan outlined in the evaluation and directs all treatment sessions toward accomplishing the goals and outcomes listed in the evaluation.

SUMMARY

The information documented in the medical record consists of:

1. Data relevant to the patient's condition
2. Problems that require medical attention
3. A treatment plan to address the problems
4. Goals of the treatment plan
5. A record of the administration of the treatments
6. Results or effectiveness of the treatment plan

The documentation content describes the medical care from the moment the patient is admitted to the moment of discharge. The information reporting the effectiveness of the treatment is the content used to determine the quality of the care provided, measure outcomes, research the most effective treatment procedures, and determine reimbursement.

A comparison of the medical diagnosis with the physical therapy diagnosis was presented. The physical therapy diagnosis is the identification of the abnormalities and dysfunctions (impairments) causing a functional limitation. The functional limitation is the primary reason the patient seeks physical therapy, and improvement of this limitation is the goal of physical therapy treatment.

Information about treatment procedures (e.g., their purposes, expected results, and any possible risks or side effects) must be explained to the patient or a representative of the patient. He or she must agree to the treatment plan before it is started. This agreement, called *informed consent,* is often made official by the patient's signing an informed consent form, which is placed in the medical record.

The documentation content is found in the written evaluation reports and the progress notes. The PT performs and writes initial, interim, and discharge examination/evaluations. The PTA can assist the PT in the examination, but does not evaluate. The PTA documents the progress notes, the focus of this book.

REFERENCES

1. American Physical Therapy Association: Guide to Physical Therapist Practice. July 1999.
2. ICIDH-2: International Classification for Functioning and Disability (Beta-2 draft, short version). World Health Organization, Geneva, 1999, p 7.
3. Goodman, CC, and Snyder, TEK: Differential Diagnosis in Physical Therapy. WB Saunders, Philadelphia, PA, 1990, p 2.
4. Sahrmann, SA: Diagnosis by the physical therapist—a prerequisite for treatment. Phys Ther 68:1703, 1988.
5. American Physical Therapy Association: Guidelines for Physical Therapy Documentation. APTA, Alexandria, VA, 1998.

➤ REVIEW EXERCISES

1. List the six categories of documentation content, and describe the content of each category.

2. Explain the difference between subjective and objective data.

3. Define signs and symptoms.

4. Compare and contrast the medical diagnosis and the physical therapy diagnosis.

5. Explain the responsibilities for documentation for the PT and PTA.

6. Describe how the PTA is involved in each of the three types of PT examination/evaluations.

7. Discuss the similarities and differences between a discharge summary and a discharge evaluation.

Practice Exercise 1 ➤ *You read in the PT initial evaluation that your patient has a fractured right femur that has healed. He is left with 2/5 strength in quadriceps and is unable to transfer independently in and out of bed or a chair.*

What is the medical problem? _____

What is the abnormality or dysfunction of the musculoskeletal system? _____

_____

What is the functional limitation? _____

Practice Exercise 2 ➤ *You read in the PT evaluation that your patient has had a cerebral vascular accident (e.g., stroke) and now has difficulty moving his left arm and leg. The PT states that the patient has weakness and extensor hypertonus in his left lower extremity with inability to ambulate stairs independently.*

What is the medical diagnosis? (pathology) _____

What is the abnormality or dysfunction of the neuromuscular system (impairment)? _____

_____

What is the functional limitation? _____

Practice Exercise 3 ➤ *You read in the PT evaluation that your patient has an incomplete spinal cord injury causing lower extremity paraparesis and inability to stand.*

What is the medical diagnosis? (pathology) _____

What is the impairment? _____

What is the functional limitation? _____

Practice Exercise 4 ➤ *Identify the documentation responsibilities of the PT and the PTA. Place "PT" next to the items that are a responsibility of the PT only. Place "PTA" next to items that are documentation tasks for the PTA.*

_____ Initial examination and evaluation

_____ Progress notes

_____ Measurement results

_____ Re-examination and re-evaluation

_____ Change in treatment plan

_____ Discharge summary with no interpretation or recommendations

_____ Discharge examination and evaluation

Identify the pathology, impairment, functional limitation, and disability after each patient description.

1. Mr. Jones, a professional football player, will never be able to play football again because he fractured a vertebra and severed his spinal cord. His legs are paralyzed and he cannot stand or walk.

   Pathology _____

   Impairment _____

   Functional limitation _____

   Disability _____

2. Sally received third-degree burns on both hands, and the scar tissue causes limited ROM in her fingers and wrists. She is unable to pick up or manipulate small objects, so she is unable to return to any work that requires fine hand manipulation.

   Pathology _____

   Impairment _____

   Functional limitation _____

   Disability _____

3. Mrs. Williams has rheumatoid arthritis with limited ROM in both knees and hips. She is unable to climb stairs or steps, so she must live and function in an environment that has no stairs or steps.

   Pathology _____

   Impairment _____

   Functional limitation _____

   Disability _____

4. Mr. Nelson's left leg was crushed in a motor vehicle accident. His leg was amputated just above his knee. He does not have the muscle strength to walk with his prosthesis (artificial leg) without the help of a cane. He will not be able to return to his old job as a railroad brakeman.

   Pathology _____

   Impairment _____

   Functional limitation _____

   Disability _____

5. Joe received a head injury in a snowmobile accident. He now has difficulty maintaining his balance when walking and frequently feels dizzy. He walks with a wheeled walker and always needs someone nearby.

Pathology _____

Impairment _____

Functional limitation _____

Disability _____

6. A little girl in the third grade has spina bifida, which has caused her legs to be very weak. She can walk independently with crutches but she cannot maintain her balance when she tries to open doors.

Pathology _____

Impairment _____

Functional limitation _____

Disability _____

Practice Exercise 6 ➤   *Place MD by the medical diagnoses, IMP by the impairments, and FL by the functional limitations.*

____ 1. Diabetes

____ 2. Rhomboid strength 3/5

____ 3. Instability

____ 4. Unable to reach top of head

____ 5. Multiple sclerosis

____ 6. Fractured neck of the femur

____ 7. Inability to walk one block

____ 8. Cannot sleep more than 3 hours

____ 9. Frequent falling

____ 10. Paralysis

____ 11. Severed ulnar nerve

____ 12. 10–90 ° knee flexion

____ 13. Cerebral palsy

____ 14. Hypermobility

____ 15. Unable to sit unsupported

(Answers are in the instructor's guide.)

Organization and Presentation of the Content

LEARNING OBJECTIVES

After studying this chapter, the student will be able to:

➤ Locate information in the medical record based on the understanding of how medical record content is organized

➤ Organize information to be documented in a physical therapy note into a logical sequence

➤ Adapt the sequence of information to three documentation models

➤ Present documentation content in at least three different formats

➤ Explain the PTA's role in Medicare documentation

INTRODUCTION

Information in the medical record communicates the story of a patient's medical care. The format used to organize information within the patient's chart varies from facility to facility. In addition, the appearance of the chart depends on the type of clinical facility. For example, the hospital medical record is different from the record used in a physical therapy private practice office. The student PTA on his or her clinical experience or the newly employed PTA should become familiar with the facility's medical record from the very beginning; the record is a good communication tool only if the reader knows where to find the information.

ORGANIZATION OF THE MEDICAL RECORD

Until the 1970s, hospitals typically used the source-oriented method for organizing the medical record. In the 1970s, the problem-oriented method was introduced, offering another way to organize information. The PTA who has the opportunity to gain work experience in several different clinical facilities may see both types of charts. More commonly, however, facilities use variations and combinations of source-oriented and problem-oriented organization. In the 21st century, the PTA may be recording in medical records organized according to the functional abilities of the patient.

Source-Oriented Medical Record

The source-oriented medical record (SOMR) is organized according to the medical services offered in the clinical facility. A section in the chart is labeled with a tab marker or color-coded for each discipline. For example, the SOMR might be organized with the physician's section first, followed by sections for nursing, physical therapy, occupational therapy, and then test results. Caregivers in each discipline document their content (e.g., data, problems, treatment plans, goals, progress notes, treatment effectiveness) in the section designated for their discipline. The sections must be clearly marked for easy identification so the reader can locate the information. Source-oriented organization is criticized because the time required to read through each section for information makes the record difficult to audit for reimbursement and quality control.

Each caregiver on the medical team should be responsible for reading the chart frequently, communicating with the other caregivers and staying informed about the patient's latest treatments and condition. One discipline might identify a patient's problem and begin treatment, whereas the rest of the disciplines may not be aware that the problem exists. For example, a nurse discovers high blood pressure and obtains medication orders from the physician. The nurse records this information in the section for nursing notes. The patient experiences side effects from this new medication that affect his or her ability to fully understand the PTA's exercise instructions. If the PTA has not taken the time to read the nursing section of the patient's chart and is unaware of this additional medication, the PTA may incorrectly assume and document that the patient is being uncooperative today, documenting this in the physical therapy section.

To ensure communication and coordination among the caregivers, regular meetings are necessary so medical personnel can gather to discuss the patient's problems and progress. A written record of these meetings should be placed in the patient's chart.

Problem-Oriented Medical Record

In the 1970s, Dr. Lawrence Weed introduced the problem-oriented medical record (POMR) as an attempt to eliminate the disadvantages associated with SOMR. Content in this type of medical record is organized around the identification and treatment of the patient's problems. The components or sections of the POMR are organized in the following sequence, thus ordering information about the patient's medical care from admission to discharge:

1. Data base
2. Problem list
3. Treatment plans
4. Progress notes
5. Discharge notes

Each section contains the appropriate information from each discipline. For example, the data gathered by the physician, PT, and occupational therapist (OT) are recorded in the data base section. For each of these disciplines, the problems identified are listed in the problem list section, the treatment plans in the treatment plan section, and the progress notes in the progress note section. Each caregiver may record on the same page within each section. Alternatively, subsections may be designated for each discipline within the main sections of the POMR.

Communication among disciplines is enhanced because the problems identified and treated by each discipline are all in one place. The organization also allows specific information, such as the treatment results, to be found easily should the record be audited.

ORGANIZATION OF THE DOCUMENTATION CONTENT

Clinical facilities commonly differ in the way documentation is organized and sequenced within the evaluation reports and progress notes. A study of some examples of content organization models reveals a common logic to the sequencing of the information.

Subjective, Objective, Assessment, Plan (SOAP) Organization

At present, the most commonly used method to organize information is the SOAP organization, developed by Dr. Weed as a component of the POMR. The SOAP writing format (SOAP is a mnemonic for Subjective, Objective, Assessment, Plan) organizes the information into a logical sequence, placing it in an outline form for quick and easy reading. "Thinking SOAP" before writing a progress note is helpful regardless of the format used because use of this mnemonic organizes the content into subjective, objective, assessment, and plan categories.

The beginnng of a SOAP-organized note may identify the discipline's diagnosis or problem the note addresses. The diagnosis or problem can be found in the problem list section of the POMR.

Subjective

The *S* section contains the subjective data; that is, information provided by the patient, his or her caregiver, a family member, or significant other. Each time the patient is seen, he or she is interviewed and questioned. This information is gathered, and these **symptoms** of the patient's disease or dysfunction are described in the subjective section.

Objective

The *O* section contains the objective data; that is, data that can be reproduced or confirmed by another professional with the same training as the person gathering the objective information. This information is gathered by measurable and reproducible tests and observations. It must be described in terms of functional movement or actions. These are the **signs** of the patient's disease or dysfunction and are recorded in the objective section. This section is a summary, "painting a picture" about the patient.

Assessment

A stands for assessment. In this section, the PT or PTA summarizes the S and O information and answers the question, "What does it mean?" In the assessment section, the PT interprets, makes a clinical judgment, and sets functional outcomes and goals based on the information in the subjective and objective sections. In the progress note, the PTA summarizes the information in the S and O sections and reports the progress being made toward accomplishing the goals. This summary also answers the "what does it mean?" question.

Plan

P stands for plan. This information describes what will happen next. The PT's treatment plan is outlined in this section of the evaluation report. In the progress note, the PTA describes what he or she may need to do before and during the next treatment session.

Examples of SOAP Organization

Suppose your 10-year-old daughter has been diagnosed by your doctor as having strep throat and an ear infection. You obtained medication and have started her on the treatment. It is the next morning.

5-18-00:   **Dx/Pr:** Strep throat and ear infection.

S: Pt. reports pain in R ear, feels too tired to go to school.

O: Temperature 100.8°F, down 2° from last night, skin color pale. Pt. sat at breakfast table 20 min before needing to lie down. Pt. took medication, 2 tablets, 8:00 AM per instructions. _____

A: Pt.'s fever decreasing but temp. not at goal of 98.6°F. Pt. is not able to stay up all day for school. _____

P: Will call attendance office to excuse pt. from school; will continue medication per Dr.'s orders.

—Super Parent, PTA

Here's another example. You are a PTA teaching a patient to walk with crutches. This patient had a skiing accident that resulted in multiple fractures of bones in the ankle joint. The ankle has been surgically treated and placed in a cast, and the patient is not permitted to bear weight on the foot.

2-16-00:   **Dx:** Fractured L ankle, repaired and casted.

PR: No weight bearing on L leg, requiring ambulation with crutches.

S: Patient states he plans to go home tomorrow and needs to climb a flight of stairs in his house and manage ramps and curbs to return to work.

O: After 3 trials requiring standby assist for sense of security and verbal cueing, patient independently ascended and descended a flight of 12 stairs using the railing (up on R, down on L) and axillary crutches, NWB on L, and independently managed a ramp and four curbs of various heights. Patient independently transferred in and out of his car, accurately following instructions.

A: Patient accomplished outcome of being able to independently manage stairs, ramps, and curbs for functioning within his house, and of community ambulation for return to work. Patient is ready for discharge.

P: Will arrange for PT discharge evaluation tomorrow.

—Alice Assistant, PTA

You can see how thinking *SOAP* organizes information so it can be documented in a logical sequence. This organization also makes it easy to find information.

Criticism of SOAP

Critics of the SOAP format state that the information focuses on the patient's impairments, implying that improvement in these will improve the patient's functional abilities. When Dr. Weed introduced the POMR and the SOAP format, documentation content did focus on the impairments (see Chapter 2). Although a SOAP-organized note can be written about functional outcomes, as seen in the crutch-walking example above, a variety of other formats are suggested, designed with a clearer focus on functional outcomes.

Problem, Status, Plan (PSP) and Problem, Status, Plan, Goals (PSPG)

A format more typically used for the progress note or interim evaluation is the PSP (mnemonic for Problem, Status, Plan), a variation of the SOAP format. The patient's physical therapy problem/diagnosis and/or medical diagnosis is stated under the first *P* section. Subjective and objective data about the patient's condition at the time of the interim evaluation are documented under *S*. The second *P* section contains the modified treatment plan indicated by the clinical findings. The PSPG format adds a *G* section for functional goals. Figures 3–1 and 3–2 are examples of notes in PSP and PSPG organization.[1]

Data, Evaluation, Performance Goals

Data, Evaluation, Performance goals (DEP), a model for performance-based documentation designed by Smith and El-Din, is another method for organizing and documenting information.[2] The subjective and objective data (D) are combined into one section. In the evaluation section (E), data is interpreted and physical therapy diagnoses are identified; the treatment plan also is included in this section. The performance goals (P) section contains the functional goals for treatment and the expected time frame for meeting these goals.

ABC Physical Therapy Clinic, Anytown, USA

June 1, 199X

P: 47 YOM, college math professor, Dx: chronic LBP syndrome; mild L spine DJD; probable lumbar extension dysfunction; r/o HNP.
S: Pt. states, "I feel 50% better. The pain in my R leg is gone now. I can sit for over an hour w/o any pain." Pt. attended back school on May 15, 199X. Exam: GMT/AROM WNL, BLE, FAROM, L spine, w/o any c/o Sx. Neg. spasm, TTP, deformity. Neg. SLR to 85° B, neg. Fabere. Gait, posture, SLT WNL. Performs extension exercises w/o difficulty or Sx.
P: Cont w/MH PRN, tid extension exercises, 10–15 reps. F/U w/ Dr. Brown scheduled for tomorrow. PT F/U 2–3 weeks or PRN. Pt. understands home program; pt. questions about exercise techniques answered._____
_____ Ron Therapist, PT

Figure 3–1 A note written in PSP organization. (From Scott, RW: Legal Aspects of Documenting Patient Care. Aspen, Gaithersburg, MD, 1994, p 79, with permission.)

Multidisciplinary Rehabilitation Center, Anytown, USA

June 1, 199X

P: 47 YOM, college math professor, Dx: chronic LBP syndrome; mild L spine DJD; probable lumbar extension dysfunction; r/o HNP.
S: Pt.was discharged as inpatient on May 5, 199X, and placed on OP home PT program of MH PRN and active extension exercises, tid X 10–15 reps. Today pt. states, "I feel 50% better. The pain in my R leg is gone. I can sit for over an hour w/o any pain." Pt. attended back school as inpatient on May 3,199X. Exam: GMT/AROM WNL, BLE. FAROM, L spine, w/o any c/o Sx. Neg. spasm, TTP, deformity, Neg. SLR to 85°B, neg. Fabere, Gait, posture, SLT WNL. Performs extension exercises w/o difficulty or Sx.
P: Cont. w/MH PRN, tid extension exercises, 10–15 reps. F/U w/Dr. Brown scheduled for tomorrow. PT F/U 2–3 wks or PRN. Pt. understands home program; pt. questions about exercise techniques answered.
G: Decrease residual Sx 50% X 2–3 wks; I pain-free ADL; prevent recurrence through good body mechanics._____
_____ Ron Therapist, PT

Figure 3–2 A note written in PSPG organization. This is a physical therapist's 4-week outpatient re-evaluation form. (From Scott, RW: Legal Aspects of Documenting Patient Care. Aspen, Gaithersburg, MD, 1994, p 79, with permission.)

Functional Outcome Report

Swanson[3] proposed the use of the functional outcome report (FOR), a structured approach for reporting functional assessment and outcomes (Box 3–1). The sequence of the information in the FOR is as follows:

1. Reason for referral
2. Functional limitations
3. Physical therapy assessment
4. Therapy problems
5. Functional outcome goals
6. Treatment plan and rationale

The reason for referral section includes the medical diagnosis, past medical history, and subjective data. The functional limitations and physical therapy assessment sections contain the objective data. The physical problems are identified based on the data. The functional goals are listed, and the report concludes with the treatment plan and how it relates to accomplishing the functional goals.

**▲ ● Box 3–1   EXAMPLE OF AN INITIAL FUNCTIONAL OUTCOME
                  REPORT**

Reason for Referral
Patient post meniscectomy of left knee reports pain, stiffness, and difficulty with walking and other upright mobility activities.

Functional Limitations

Activity	Current Status
Sit-to-stand transfer	Independent
Standing balance	Performs independently, with cane
Flat terrain ambulation (speed)	Performs with cane for more than 18 sec for 20 ft
Flat terrain ambulation (endurance)	Tolerates less than 5 min
Ambulation on uneven terrain	Unable
Stair climbing	Ascends two steps, descends two steps with railing and minimum assistance

PT Assessment
Medical diagnosis status post meniscectomy is further defined to include residual left knee joint inflammation.
Positive test findings: Positive fluctuation test; limited strength; quadriceps 3/5 and hamstring 4/5, indicative of synovial effusion.

Therapy Problems
1. Pain on compression maneuvers of the left knee: sitting, sit to stance, periodically during gait cycle, during all phases of stair climbing.
2. Difficulty in coordinating gait cycle with use of cane to reduce stress to left knee.

Functional Outcome Goals

Activity	Performance	Due Date
Flat terrain ambulation (speed)	Independent without device; 20 ft in 9 sec	Within 14 days
Flat terrain ambulation (endurance)	Tolerates unassisted walking for 30 min	Within 21 days
Uneven terrain ambulation	Tolerates for a minimum of 15 min	Within 14 days
Stair climbing	Ascends and descends 15 steps	Within 21 days

Treatment Plan with Rationale
Application of anti-inflammatory modalities with instruction for follow-up home program to minimize post-activity edema.
Lower extremity strength training with instruction in progressive home exercise program.
Patient instructed in activity limits and restrictions during the course of care.

From Swanson, G: Functional Outcome Report: The next generation in physical therapy reporting. In Steward, D, and Abein, S (eds). Documenting Functional Outcomes in Physical Therapy. Mosby Yearbook, St. Louis, MO, 1993.

LOGICAL SEQUENCING OF CONTENT

All of the content organization models previously discussed use a problem-solving approach to sequence the information. First, the data are gathered. Second, the data are interpreted and a judgment is made to identify the physical therapy diagnosis. Next, goals and outcomes are determined to direct the focus of physical therapy interventions. Finally, treatment plans designed to accomplish the goals and outcomes are outlined. Table 3–1 compares the organization models for similarities and their methods of incorporating documentation content.

Guidelines for Adapting to the Organization Formats

The PTA can easily adapt to any format of documentation for the progress note by using the following problem-solving approach to sequence the information:

1. Introduce the progress note with a list or statement that tells the reader the physical therapy diagnoses about which the note is written.
2. Place the subjective and objective data first. Compare it with or relate it to the data in the initial or interim examination report.
3. Discuss the meaning of the data as it relates to treatment effectiveness and progress toward accomplishing the goals and functional outcomes listed in the initial or interim evaluation report.
4. Discuss the plan for future treatment sessions and involvement of the PT.

This organization is illustrated in the following progress note about the student injured in a motorcycle accident (see Chapter 2):

6-27-00: **Dx:** Status post pinned fractured R femur.

PT Dx: Dependent ambulation because of NWB on R leg.

Patient states he feels dizzy when he sits up but is eager to start walking on crutches and go home. Pt. c/o dizziness first time standing during treatment. Blood pressure before treatment 120/70 mmHg, first time up in // bars 108/65 mmHg, second standing trial 118/70 mmHg, after treatment 128/72 mmHg. Pt. responded to gait training with axillary crutches/minimal assist for sense of security and verbal cues for posture and heel contact/NWB on R/swing through gait 100 ft 2× in hall, bed ↔ bathroom, and on carpet. Able to ① sit ↔ stand with crutches from bed/lounge chair/toilet. Pt.'s progress toward functional outcome of community ambulation with crutches 50%. Blood pressure adjusting to upright position. Will teach stairs, ambulation on grass, and car transfers tomorrow AM. Will notify PT discharge evaluation scheduled for tomorrow PM.

—Connie Competent, PTA Lic. #7890

FORMATS FOR THE PRESENTATION OF THE CONTENT

Information can be recorded using a variety of formats. Evaluations and progress notes may be handwritten or dictated and typed. The progress notes may be narrative (i.e., written in paragraph form) or written in an outline format such as the SOAP note. How the information in the medical record is organized depends on the preference of the medical facility. Each facility decides the format to use for recording data. The PTA must be familiar with the facility's charting procedures and must always follow the facility's policies, procedures, and format.

Table 3–1 ► COMPARING ORGANIZATION MODELS

Documentation content	SOAP	DEP	PSPG	FOR
Problem	Pr	D	P	Current therapy diagnoses
Subjective data	S	D	S	Functional limitations
				Current status
Objective data	O	D	S	Functional limitations
				Current status
Treatment effectiveness	A	E	S	Functional limitations
				Current status
Goals/outcomes	A	P	G	Functional outcome goals
Plan	P	E	P	Treatment plan with rationale

A = Assessment, D = Data, E = Evaluation, G = Goals, O = Objective data, P = Plan in SOAP and performance in DEP, Pr = Problem, S = Subjective data in SOAP and Status in PSPG

Computerized Documentation

Currently available computer software programs are designed for writing evaluations and progress notes. Many facilities have one or more computers in the department for the staff to use when documenting. A few facilities do have a computer terminal in every hospital room or in all the treatment areas of a physical therapy department. This allows the caregiver to enter information in the patient's chart immediately after treatment. Physical therapy documentation software is advertised in publications such as *Physical Therapy* and *PT Magazine.*

A word of warning is necessary about computerized documentation. The chapters in Part Two of this text discuss how the content of the progress note must be individualized to each patient, to clearly demonstrate how each patient is responding to the physical therapy intervention/treatment plan. Computerized documentation programs typically have preprogrammed statements or phrases that can be selected and combined to quickly compose the content of the progress note. The PTA must be careful that the selection of these phrases will clearly distinguish this patient from other patients, and that the content will clearly describe the necessity for providing skilled physical therapy services. The software should allow the writer to type in his or her own words and phrases to individualize the note.

Flow Charts and Checklists

Much of the data, such as vital signs, physical therapy interventions provided, and the patient's functional status, can be recorded on flow charts, fill-in-the-blank forms, and checklists. Using these formats, the caregiver can record in the chart quickly and easily. The reader also can easily visually scan the form to gather the information. Hospitals, long-term care facilities, and rehabilitation centers are facilities where the PTA will find narrative or outlined (commonly SOAP) notes, checklists, and flow charts. Figure 3–3 is an example of a flow chart for recording physical therapy treatments. Figure 3–4 on pages 36 and 37 illustrates two progress note forms combining checklists and flow charts with brief statements and narration. A fill-in-the-blank form is depicted in Figure 3–5 on page 38.

Letter Format

Physical therapists in private practice may communicate information about the patient to other caregivers by letter. The data are recorded in the office by any of the models already mentioned, but they are periodically summarized in letter format. This type of format is commonly used when the patient's progress is being reported to a physician.

Individual Educational Program

In the public schools, physical therapy, occupational therapy, speech therapy, and psychologic services provided to a student are planned and recorded in a format called an individual educational program (IEP). This format is in accordance with several laws passed by Congress relating to the provision of services to facilitate the education of students with disabilities. Professionals representing these services (e.g., teacher, OT, PT, school psychologist, speech pathologist) are included on the IEP team. The team records educational goals and objectives to be accomplished during the school year and holds meetings periodically to review the goals and objectives. It also meets with parents a minimum of every 6 months to make any needed changes. Box 3–2 on page 38 lists the components of an IEP. These components are essentially the same as those of the physical therapy evaluation and progress note content. Figure 3–6 on page 39 is an example of the PT's contribution to the annual long-term goals and instructional objectives in an IEP written for a student. The PTA does not write the physical therapy goals and objectives for the IEP but plays an important role by providing input for their planning. The PTA working in the school environment will document the progress being made toward accomplishing the physical therapy goals.

Cardex

Within the physical therapy department, the patient's treatment goals and current intervention plan may be recorded in a cardex format. This 4″ × 6″ card is kept in a folder designed to hold many cards for quick access. The information is written in pencil so it can be updated easily. For example, in the morning the card may read that the patient ambulates from his bedroom to the nursing station and ambulates on the carpet in the lounge area. However, during the treatment session later in the afternoon, the patient ambulated past the station and to the stairs. The patient also managed three stairs for the first time. Now the information needs to be erased, and the new ambulation distance and the stair climbing must be described. When the PTA is treating a patient, he or she refers to the cardex information. Updating the information

DATE:

Orientation/Mood						
UE Strength/Ex — bicep/tricep						
— W/C push up/rowing						
— shld flex/abd/horz abd/add						
TRANSPORT:						
— transport to dept W/C/cart/amb						
Abductor pillow/knee immobilizer/prothesis/tilt tbl.						
— standing table						
GAIT: DEVICE:						
//bars; walker; crutches; cane; Qcane; none						
wt. bearing: NWB; TTWB; PWB; FWB; WBAT						
pattern: 2pt./3pt./4pt.						
distance/endurance						
Balance - sit/stand/walk						
Balance Act: lat/post/braid/line/sit/ball						
Stairs: rail/without rail/gait sequence						
TF's bed mobility						
toilet/raised seat/reg/commode bedside						
slidingboard transfer						
shower seat/car transfers						
supine--> sit; sit --> supine/sit to stand						
EX isometric quad, glut, HS, abd/ball squeeze						
ankle pump/circle/TB DF/PF/Ev/Inv						
hip flexion supine/sit/stand						
SLR flexion supine/stand						
SLR extension prone/stand/side lie						
SLR abduction supine/side lie/stand						
TKE supine/sit/SAQ/LAQ						
Bridging 1 leg/both						
knee AAROM sit/prone/supine						
KA PROM hip/knee/UE/ankle						
AAROM hip/knee/UE/ankle						
Stretching LE/UE						
Positional ROM/prone/long sit						
CPM						
Modalities H.P./ice/US/whirlpool						
Neuromusc. Re-Educ. Biofeed/CVA rehab						
HHA/Family instruction in:						
TF's-bed/toilet/shower/chair						
positioning/EX program						
walking program						
Written home program provided						
CHARGE - abbreviation for treatment						
THERAPIST						

SPC 337022   **REHABILITATION PHYSICAL THERAPY**

Restraints: NA / pelvic / vest

DNR   Y / N

Precautions:_____

Figure 3–3   Flow chart form for recording physical therapy treatments.

on a regular basis is essential to ensure that the patient is progressing toward accomplishing the treatment goals. This cardex is to be used within the PT department; it is not a part of the patient's medical record. An intervention plan outlined on a cardex is depicted in Figure 3–7 on page 40.

Standardized Medicare Forms

Standardized Medicare forms are used to chart the medical care given to patients covered by Medicare. The Health Care Financing Administration specifies the format and the time lines for recording and submitting data. The Medicare Updated Plan of Progress for Rehabilitation form (FORM HCFA-701), a recertification form (see Fig. 3–8 on p. 41), is intended to be an evaluation form. This form should not be completed by a PTA.

The approval for physical therapy services is periodically renewed or recertified (at present, every 30 days). When the PT recommends that therapy be continued for the patient to meet the goals, this form becomes an interim evaluation. If the patient has reached maximum benefit or has met the goals, this form serves as a discharge evaluation. The PTA can provide the PT with information about the status of the patient, but the PT completes the form.

(text continued on page 42)

PHYSICAL THERAPY PROGRESS NOTES
HOME CARE / HOSPICE
SERVICES

Patient's Name:	Last		First		Age	Date	Time	Visit Frequency	Date Next Visit
Mood		Orientation		Cooperation		Communication		Pain	RX Tolerance

TREATMENTS			COMMENTS	
Modalities	**WB Status**	**Ambulation**	**Exercise:**	
Bed mobility	Non wt. bearing	Distance		
Elec. stim.	Partial	Assist.		
Ex. active	Toe touch	Balance		
Ex ROM	Full	Coord.		
Ex back	Non amb.	Pattern		
Ex breathing		Stairs		
Ex coord.				
Ex isometric	**Equipment**	**Transfers**	**Problems/Progress:**	
Ex man. resist	Walker	Bed		
Ex mm re-ed.	Crutches	Toilet		
Ex PRE	Cane	Tub		
Ex gait trng.		Chair		
Massage		Car		
Packs	**ROM**			
Stump wrap				
Transfers		Other		
Tx				
Ultrasound				
Evaluation				
MD contact				
Instruction		**Follow-through/Response:**		
Patient				
Support Person				
HHA				

THERAPIST SIGNATURE

7400-17-11/93

Figure 3–4 Progress note forms that combine presentation styles. The form on this page combines a checklist with brief statements. The form on the facing page combines a flow chart with narration.

(continued on next page)

MODALITIES:	DATE/Initials	DATE/Initials	DATE/Initials	DATE/Initials	DATE/Initials	DATE/Initials
Hot Pack/Cold Packs						
Massage/Ice Massage						
Electrical Stimulation						
Traction						
Ultrasound						
Kinetic Activity						
Therapeutic Exercise						
Neuromuscular Re-ed						
Functional Activities						
Training in ADL's						
Serial Casting						
Gait Training						
Orthotics/Prosthetics Train.						
Wound Care						
Whirlpool Therapy						
Conference						
Consultation						
Other						

Date	Comments:

Assessment:

Goals:

Plan:

(Name)	Date
(Name)	Date
(Name)	Date

Treatment Diagnosis:

P120 NEW 7/94

Physical Therapy Daily Progress Notes

Figure 3–4 Continued.

ACTIVITIES OF DAILY LIVING:

Level of Independence	Without Help	Uses Device	Help of Another	Device & Help	Dependent/ Does Not Do	Not Determined
Feeding						
Hygiene/Groom-ing						
Transfers						
Homemaking						
Bath/Shower						
Dressing						
Bed Mobility						
Home Mgmt						

Physical Environment: _____

_____

Psychosocial: _____

*Safety Measures: _____

_____

Equipment in Home: _____
Emergency No: _____ *Nutritional Req:_____ Allergies: _____
Unusual Home/Social Environment: _____
*Known Medical Reason Pt. leaves home: _____
Other Services Involved: _____ *Prognosis: _____
Vulnerable Adult Assessment: _____Low Risk   _____High Risk
Caregiver Status: _____
Pulse _____   BP _____

Current Medications : _____   _____

                      _____   _____

                      _____   _____

Patient's Prior Status: _____

_____

Scheduled MD Follow-up appt (s): _____

_____

Name_____
R# _____

Figure 3–5   Figure 3–5 Form with a fill-in-the-blank format.

▲

● **Box 3–2   COMPONENTS OF AN IEP**

1. A statement of the student's current levels of educational performance.
2. A statement of annual goals, including short-term instructional objectives.
3. A statement of the specific special education and related services to be provided to the student and the extent to which the child will be able to participate in regular education programs.
4. The projected dates for initiation of services and the anticipated duration of the services.
5. Appropriate objective criteria and evaluation procedures and schedules for determining on at least an annual basis, whether the short-term instructional objectives are being achieved (34CFR 300.334).

From American Physical Therapy Association and the Section on Pediatrics: Individualized educational program and individualized family service plan. In Martin, KD (ed): Physical Therapy Practice in Educational Environments: Policies and Guidelines. APTA, Alexandria, VA. 1990, p. 6.1.

Learner's Name: _____

ANNUAL GOALS, SHORT-TERM INSTRUCTIONAL OBJECTIVES

Thoroughly state the goal. List objectives for the goal, including attainment criteria for each objective.	GOAL# _____ OF _____ GOALS

GOAL:
The student will independently move about the school building and within the classroom using a wheelchair to participate in all daily school activities, and the student will independently transfer from wheelchair to desk seat, to floor for participation and position change in 6 months.

Short-Term Instructional Objectives

1. The student will independently open doors to the gymnasium and maneuver the wheelchair through the entrance to the gym 1 out of 3 trials in 3 months.

2. The student will independently transfer from wheelchair to floor and back into the chair 1 out of 3 trials in 3 months.

3. The student will safely and independently maneuver the wheelchair around the tables in the cafeteria 1 out of 3 trials in 3 months.

G.   IEP PERIODIC REVIEW

Date Reviewed: _____   Progress made toward this goal and objective

The learner's IEP

☐ Meets learner's current needs and will be continued without changes.

☐ Does not meet learner's current needs and the modifications (not significant) listed below will be made without an IEP meeting unless you contact us.

☐ Does not meet learner's current needs and the significant changes listed below require a revised IEP. We will be in contact soon to schedule a meeting.

NOTE TO PARENT(S): You are entitled to request a meeting to discuss the results of this review.

Figure 3–6 An example of the PT's contribution to the goals and instructional objectives on an individual educational program (IEP) written for a child in the school.

| DX: R CVA with L hemiplegia | | | | | INITIAL DATE: 2-24-00 |
| PRECAUTIONS: Broca's Aphasia, feeding tube | | | | | UPDATE: 3-20-00 |

Exercise	Set	Rep	Equipment	Assist	Goals
PROM/AAROM L UE & L LE	1	10		muscle belly	1. Independent bed mobility
PRE R UED1 & D2 diagonals, supine	1	10	1# cuff wt	tapping	2. Independent unsupported sitting
	1	10	2# cuff wt	verbal cues	3. Independent wheelchair mobility
	1	as many as he can, goal 10 reps			4. Standing pivot transfer with minimum assist of 1
Resistive active exercise R LE					
SLR, abduction sidelying, prone knee flexion	2	10	2# cuff wt	verbal cues	
TKE long sitting	2	10	1# cuff wt standing table		TDD:
Standing 10 min; work on eye tracking and mouth closure					TDP:

Patient's Name	Age	Sex	MD	PT	RM#	Units
Harry A	71	M	Smith	Jones	E123	12

Transfers bed <–> w/c, w/c <–> mat table, w/c <–> toilet, w/c <–> straight chair	Method stand pivot to R side	Assist maximum x1	Other Practice squat pivot transfer w/c <–> mat moving towards L

Pregait/Gait
Stand in // bars - max assist x1 - midline with mirror and wt shifting to L. Watch L knee - no hyperextension.
Sitting balance in w/c with arms removed and in armless straight chair. Minimum assist x2. Work on head movement, eye tracking, wt shifting, trunk rot.
W/c mobility - room to bathroom, room to dining room, to PT department, to OT, speech. Check seating/cushion, L scapula protracted, arm on tray.

Figure 3–7   A treatment plan outlined on a cardex, commonly used in physical therapy departments to keep treatment procedures current.

DEPARTMENT OF HEALTH AND HUMAN SERVICES
HEALTH CARE FINANCING ADMINISTRATION

FORM APPROVED
OMB NO. 0938-0227

UPDATED PLAN OF PROGRESS FOR OUTPATIENT REHABILITATION
(Complete for Interim to Discharge Claims. Photocopy of HCFA-700 or 701 is required)

1. PATIENT'S LAST NAME	FIRST NAME	M.I.	2. PROVIDER NO.	3. HICN

4. PROVIDER NAME	5. MEDICAL RECORD NO. *(Optional)*	6. ONSET DATE 8-1-95	7. SOC. DATE

8. TYPE: ☒ PT ☐ OT ☐ SLP ☐ CR ☐ RT ☐ PS ☐ SN ☐ SW

9. PRIMARY DIAGNOSIS *(Pertinent Medical D.X.)* ℞ CVA

10. TREATMENT DIAGNOSIS ℞ paraparesis dep, bed mob transfer ambulation

11. VISITS FROM SOC.

12. FREQ/DURATION (e.g., 3/Wk x 4 Wk) 6x/wk x 8 wks

13. CURRENT PLAN UPDATE, FUNCTIONAL GOALS *(Specify changes to goals and plan)*

GOALS (Short Term) 1. 3-4/5 strength ② UE/LE for 4-8 wks ① bed mob transfers SBA, min A amb
2. SBA bed mob 4 wks ① 8 wks
3. min A transfer bed↔chair↔toilet 4 wks STBA 8 wks 4. Amb/quad cane/carpeting 100' mod A 4 wks, 300' min A 8 wk

OUTCOME (Long Term) Return to home with wife ① in bed mob SBA transfers + min A ambulation in home

PLAN 1. Strengthening exs
2. ② dorsiflexion re-education
3. Bed mob, transfer training
4. Balance activities
5. Gait training

I HAVE REVIEWED THIS PLAN OF TREATMENT AND RECERTIFY A CONTINUING NEED FOR SERVICES. ☐ N/A ☐ DC

14. RECERTIFICATION FROM 9-8-95 THROUGH 10-8-95 ☐ N/A

15. PHYSICIAN'S SIGNATURE   16. DATE   17. ON FILE (Print/type physician's name) ☐

18. REASON(S) FOR CONTINUING TREATMENT THIS BILLING PERIOD *(Clarify goals and necessity for continued skilled care)*

Pt. has met 4 wk STG for bed mobility and transfers. Requires more training for safety measures due to left side neglect and for techniques to overcome "freezing" caused by Parkinson's. Further balance and gait training needed with new AFO. Muscle re-education should be continued for ② ankle dorsiflexion for safe ambulation with min A. Expect pt. to be d/c to home in 4 wks requiring min A from wife for ambulating on carpet in the home.

19. SIGNATURE (or name of professional, including prof. designation) Marianne Lukas, PT

20. DATE 9-6-95

21. ☒ CONTINUE SERVICES OR ☐ DC SERVICES

22. FUNCTIONAL LEVEL (at end of billing period - Relate your documentation to functional outcomes and list problems still present)

1. Pt ① in all bed mobility activities
2. Pt performs transfers bed↔chair↔toilet with min A for controlling ② ankle and safety cues.
3. Pt ambulates with a quad cane + ② AFO, 100' on tile with mod A for balance + wt shifting when bringing ② LE through. Pt requires mod A on carpeting for balance and advancing ② LE.
4. General muscle strength in ② UE/LE except ② ankle 3/5.
5. ② ankle dorsiflexion 3/5.
6. Complicating factors: ②-side neglect and Parkinson's Disease

23. SERVICE DATES FROM 8-11-95 THROUGH 9-8-95

FORM HCFA-701 (11-91)

Figure 3–8 A Medicare recertification form.

SUMMARY   Information in the medical chart is organized according to the source of the medical services provided (SOMR), the patient's problems (POMR), or combinations and variations of these two types. Each health-care discipline has a section in the SOMR. The POMR sections consist of the database, problem list, treatment plans, and progress and discharge notes.

Documentation content is organized into a logical sequence: Typically, data are listed first. They are followed by the interpretation and relevance of the data to the patient's functional abilities and goals, and finally the treatment plans are identified. A variety of formats, such as SOAP, DEP, PSPG, or FOR, may be used for organizing the content. The PTA must be able to adapt to effectively use the type of format preferred by the facility.

Information in the medical record is recorded in a variety of formats. Notes are written in a narrative paragraph or in a SOAP outline. Flow charts, graphs, checklists, and fill-in-the-blank forms are often used in hospitals and rehabilitation centers, whereas private practice therapists may put the information into a letter to the physician. In schools, the child's treatment plan and goals are incorporated into an IEP. Medicare information is documented on standardized Medicare forms.

REFERENCES   1. Scott, RW: Legal Aspects of Documenting Patient Care. Aspen, Gaithersburg, MD, 1994.
2. El-Din, D, and Smith, GJ: Performance Based Documentation: A Tool for Functional Documentation, Preconference workshop. APTA CSM, February 1995, Reno, NV.
3. Swanson, G: Functional outcome report: The next generation in physical therapy reporting. In Stewart, D, and Abeln, S (eds): Documenting Functional Outcomes in Physical Therapy. Mosby–Year Book, St. Louis, MO, 1993.
4. American Physical Therapy Association and the Section on Pediatrics: Individualized educational program and individualized family service plan. In Martin, KD (ed): Physical Therapy Practice in Educational Environments: Policies and Guidelines. APTA, Alexandria, VA, 1990, p. 6.1.

➤ REVIEW EXERCISES

1. Explain how the SOMR and the POMR differ.

2. Describe the information documented in each section of a SOAP-organized note.

3. Define PSPG, DEP, and FOR.

4. Discuss how the PTA can adapt to any model for organizing documentation content.

5. List three formats in which documentation content may be presented, and identify the types of physical therapy facilities most likely to use each format.

6. Discuss the PTA's role in Medicare recertification documentation.

7. Documentation procedures are different in each physical therapy clinic. What rule should the PTA follow?

Practice Exercise 1 ▶

Think of two events that occurred recently in your life (e.g., car problem and how you solved it, lost keys and how they were found), and write about them in SOAP format. Organize the information so what is told to you (subjective data) is in the S section, measurable happenings and things you observed (objective data) are in the O section, the meaning of or your conclusions about the data are in the A section, and what you plan to do next is in the P section.

Write one of your notes in outline form using SOAP headings, as in the notes on pages 29 and 30. Write one of the notes in paragraph form with the information sequenced in SOAP organization, but with no headings. _____

_____

_____

_____

Practice Exercise 2 ▶

You have treated your patient and have taken notes about the treatment session. Arrange your notes so they are in a logical sequence in preparation for writing your progress note. You may want to refer to the guidelines on page 33.

Outcome ① sit to stand met.

Observed patient sitting in middle of couch.

Patient expresses frustration can't get up from couch without help, especially in evening.

Dx: Multiple sclerosis.

Gross MMT 32/5 all LE muscle groups, 2/5 initial eval.

PT Dx: LE weakness limiting ability to sit ↔ stand and ambulate safely.

Patient sat at end of couch, scooted forward to edge, used couch arm to help push up. 3rd trial able to sit to stand ① Verbal cues to lean forward.

Instructed patient not to sit on couch in evening when fatigued and weaker.

Strength gain LEs.

Will visit patient 2 more times and schedule PT discharge evaluation.

Practice Exercise 3 ▶

Rewrite this unorganized note so the information flows in a logical order. Refer to the guidelines on page 33.

3-26-00
_____

Pt. has met his short-term outcome of ① crutch walking on level and uneven ground. Says he needs to be able to climb three flights of stairs to get to his apartment. Will work on stair climbing next session. Handrail on L going up. Pt. ambulated, NWB R, axillary crutches, ①, on grass and uneven sidewalk, 300 ft R ankle & foot edema. Circumference equals L foot & ankle measurements (see initial eval). All R ankle AROM WNL, R knee flexion PROM 10–110° (15–100° last session). Pt. correctly demonstrated self knee ROM & gentle stretching exercises (see copy in chart). RLE mobility progressing. Will inform PT pt. will be ready for discharge evaluation next session. Limited RLE mobility and NWB because of Fx R femur, pinned 3-22-00.

—Confused Student, SPTA/Puzzled Therapist, PT (Lic. #420)

_____

_____

_____

_____

_____

Practice Exercise 4 ➤ *Rearrange the following notes taken during the treatment session so they are in a logical order in preparation for writing the progress note. Follow the guidelines for adapting to the various formats for organizing content.*

Sam Smart, PTA lic #007

Patient c/o itching around wound.

6/10/00

Wound healing as diameter is 2 cm smaller than at initial treatment.

During gait training, pt. ① ambulated with axillary crutches, toe-touch gait pattern for left, on grass, curbs, sidewalk, carpeting, in/out car, stairs.

Good posture, good step-through gait.

Whirlpool/105°F/sitting/left heel/to remove dressings/10 min

Outcome for independent ambulation in home and community met.

Will report to PT re d/c gait training.

Will continure wound care per POC.

Diameter wound 4 cm (6 cm initial treatment).

Teaspoon drainage, clear, no odor.

Wound pink.

Goal for healed wound 50% met.

Patient says feels comfortable and safe on cruthes.

Sterile dressings applied per previous treatment procedures.

(Answer in the instructor's guide)

You have been treating your patient who had a R CVA with L hemiplegia, following the treatment plan on the cardex (see Fig. 3–7). Your patient has progressed and the cardex needs to be updated, especially because you will be on vacation next week and another PTA will be seeing your patient. The changes include the following: 5 reps active assistive L scapular protraction in supine with active assistive elbow extension facilitated by tapping triceps muscle belly, RUE PREs 2 lb, 10×/3 lb, 10×/4 lb as many reps as can (stop at 10), 5-lb cuff wts., for all RLE exercises, ambulation in // bars 2× with max. assist of 2 to facilitate wt. shift to L and control knee, using temporary AFO on L ankle, sitting balance now min. assist of 1, now ① with w/c mobility as brings self to therapy. Standing table discontinued. Other LUE exercises the same.

Write in the changes and update the cardex below.

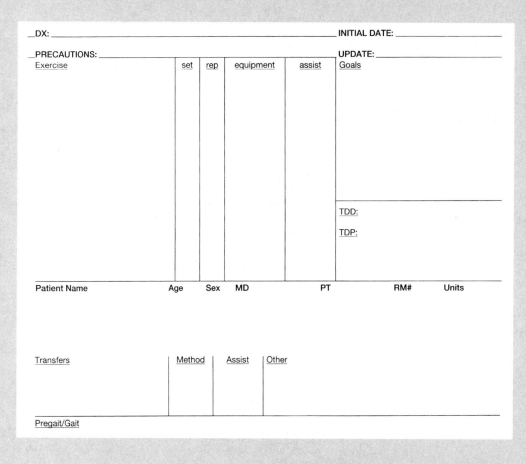

You are a PTA working on the orthopedic floor at the local hospital. You are treating Earl, a 62-year-old farmer, who has just had R total knee arthroplasty surgery, and the PT saw him on day 1 postoperation. The discharge goals are (1) independent ambulation on tiling, carpeting, stairs, and inclines with the least restrictive and most appropriate assistive device; and (2) independent transfers. Active knee ROM should be 90° at discharge. Treatments are to include CPM, 1 hour on/1 hour off until 70° is reached; isometric exercises for quads, gluts, hamstrings; ankle pumps; TKE; SLR; and active knee flexion. Gait training is to start on day 2 in the AM. A cold pack/ice pack may be used on the knee as needed.

Document the following treatment sessions on the flow sheet on the next page.

Day 2: All isometrics independent with good coordination. CPM increased to 40°. Active knee flexion while supine 3–30°. Bed mobility transfers (supine to sit) mod. assist of one to support knee. Unable to do SLR independently. In sitting, still requires support to R knee as pain too severe for initiation of ROM exercises. Ice pack to knee almost continuous. Drain in place for AM session; removed by PM session. Able to stand at side of bed, PWB RLE. Did not attempt ambulation because of pain.

Day 3: AM: Able to sit at side of bed with AROM to 45°, much pain. BP 140/85 mmHg, pulse at 72 BPM before standing. Stood at side of bed with mod. assist of one, PWB to approx. 50% of body weight on RLE, used walker. Took several steps to chair, then sat. Uses standing pivot transfer with walker. BP 145/88 mmHg, pulse 100 BPM. Independent with all exercises. Supine knee flexion to 35°. CPM to 60° PM as in AM, but able to ambulate 50 ft 1× with walker, PWB at 50% body weight. Continues to keep ice pack on knee.

Day 4: AM: Ambulated 50 ft 2× with walker on level surface, tile, and carpet. Sitting AROM 60°, CPM increased to 70°. Supine AROM 5–55° flexion. Min. assist with SLR. PM: ambulated 50 ft 2× with walker, SBA. Ambulated 60 ft 1× with crutches on level, min. assist of one. Remains PWB with up to 75% body weight. AROM sitting to 75°, supine 5–60°. SBA for supine to sit transfer, independent transfer sit to stand. Independent with SLR. Ice pack discontinued this morning.

Day 5: AM: Independent with all exercises and all standing pivot transfers. CPM discontinued last night by nursing. Ambulates independently 125 ft with crutches, 3-point step through gait on tile and carpeting. SBA on stairs and inclines. Knee ROM sitting to 85°, supine 5–80°. PT to see patient in PM for discharge evaluation.

TOTAL KNEE ARTHROPLASTY									
	Date 8-8-00		Date		Date		Date		Date
	am	pm	am	pm	am	pm	am	pm	am pm
CPM Degrees	25	25							
CPM Time	1 hr on/1 hr off								
Knee ROM AA = Active Assist A = Active Supine									
Sitting									
Exercises: Isometrics Quads/Gluts/HS									
Ankle Pumps									
TKE									
SLR									
Active Knee Flex									
Transfers: Bed Mobility									
Toilet/Commode									
Shower Seat									
Car Transfer									
Standing Pivot									
Sliding Board									
Supine <--> Sit									
Sit <--> Stand									
Balance: Sitting									
Standing									
Ambulation: Device									
Weight Bearing									
Pattern									
Distance									
Surface									
Assist									
Stairs									
Blood Pressure									
Pulse									
Modalities	ice pack prn								
THERAPIST	Jennifer Nice, PT								

PHYSICAL THERAPY PROGRESS

PRECAUTIONS: Drain in place 8-8-00

NAME: Earl

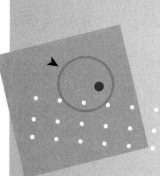

Part Two

How to Document

Writing the Content: Guidelines

LEARNING OBJECTIVES

After studying this chapter, the student will be able to:
➤ Discuss the use of the progress note in the medical record
➤ Describe two formats for presenting progress note information
➤ List the guidelines for documenting in a legal record
➤ Read sample progress notes, identifying the legal guidelines that were not followed

INTRODUCTION

The first three chapters discussed the definition and purpose of documentation, identified the categories of content documented in the medical record, and presented a variety of formats for organizing content. The next five chapters focus on the actual writing of the content. The guidelines, instructions, and suggestions focus on the progress note written by the PTA.

THE PROGRESS NOTE

In the medical record, the progress notes are the record of the treatment procedures or interventions administered. In the physical therapy chart, they are the written report of the patient's physical therapy treatment sessions. The information in progress notes provides proof that the treatment plan outlined in the initial evaluation report is appropriate, is being carried out, and is effective; it documents a treatment progression focused on accomplishing the goals and outcomes established in the initial evaluation report. Thus, important supportive evidence is available for the purpose of reimbursement and quality assurance.

Writing Frequency

The frequency of the documentation is influenced by the requirements of the insurance company, the documentation standards the facility must follow, and the facility's policies. Usually, the progress note is written after each treatment session or after a series of sessions. However, the more acute the patient's condition is, the more frequently the progress notes are written. Typically, progress notes are documented less frequently with chronic conditions. PTs and PTAs usually document daily or weekly.

Content and Form

According to the American Physical Therapy Association's (APTA) *Guidelines for Physical Therapy Documentation,*[1] continuum-of-care documentation should include identification of specific interventions provided; equipment provided; and patient/client status, progress, or regression. The note should state specifically what was done during the treatment session and the functional outcome.

In most facilities the notes are written in either narrative form or SOAP (subjective, objective, assessment, and plan) outline. However, the information may be in other similar formats such as the DEP (data, evaluation, performance goals), FOR (functional outcome report), or PSPG (problem, status, plan, goals) (see Chapter 3). Many use formats that combine descriptive information with flow sheets, checklist forms, or graphs and charts. Figure 4–1 illustrates a PTA progress note written as a narrative or paragraph organized in the SOAP format.

Medical and Physical Therapy Diagnosis

The diagnosis and the problem may introduce the progress note in the medical record, as illustrated in Figures 4–1 and 4–2. Not all facilities use this format, but the PTA may see this in a POMR (problem-oriented medical record). When the problems are listed and numbered on the problem list in the POMR, then the number of the problem or diagnosis being documented is placed in the margin or at the heading of the note. In many facilities, the problems are not numbered.

Example:
1. **Dx:** Multiple sclerosis
   PT Dx: #2: Ataxia of lower extremities causing frequent falling.
2. **Dx:** Fractured right femur
   PT Dx: 2/5 strength of quadriceps limiting ability to independently move from sitting to standing.

PRINCIPLES FOR DOCUMENTING IN A LEGAL RECORD

Following the principles and guidelines for documenting in the legal record will provide the PTA with a good start toward quality care and documentation. The guidelines for documenting in the medical record are incorporated into each facility's documentation standards. Again, the best rule is to follow the facility's procedures.

Always document with the assumption that the information will be read by lawyers and jurors in court. When writing in a medical record, think, "Dear ladies and gentlemen of the jury."[2] This will remind the PTA that the medical record is a legal document and, therefore, that guidelines described below must be followed.

Accuracy

"*Never* record falsely, exaggerate, or make up data." (p 8).[3] Information that is pertinent to the patient's care should never be omitted, even if it might be damaging to the PTA. The court is more likely to be lenient when all information is recorded in the medical record and a mistake is admitted.[2] Keep information relevant to the patient.

5-18-00   **Dx:** Fx R hip.
PT Dx: Dependent ambulation 2° Fx R hip.
Pt. states his hip feels sore today but not painful; feels he should be able to walk better. Pt. ambulated bed to dining room (330 ft) with min. assist for loss of balance recovery 2X, standard walker, partial weight-bearing on right. Posture erect, pt. looks ahead. Quality of pt.'s gait & balance improved (see 5-16-00 note), making good progress toward goal of independent ambulation. Continue ambulation training per PT initial plan. Will teach stair climbing next session and add ambulation on carpet.

Jane Doe, PTA (Lic. #)

Figure 4–1   A PTA progress note is written as a narrative or paragraph organized in SOAP format.

> **9-12-00** AM **Dx:** L hip fracture.
> **PT Dx:** Dependent with pivot transfer.
> **S:** Patient states she pivoted chair <---> bed with minimal help from daughter last night. _____
> **O:** 9-12-00 ss. After three trials, pt. stood & pivoted non–weight-bearing on left, chair <—> mat, WC <—> toilet, bed <—> WC with SBA for loss of balance recovery if needed. No loss of balance. _____
> **A:** Pt. ready for pivot transfer with SBA with nursing. Making good progress toward goal of independent transfers. _____
> **P:** Will notify PT & nursing.
>
> Sally Student, SPTA/Mary Therapist, PT (Lic. #)

Figure 4–2   An example of a progress note following legal guidelines.

Brevity   State information in short, concise sentences. Keep the note brief by staying focused on the information relevant to the effectiveness of the treatment and changes and improvement in the patient's functional abilities. Abbreviations should be avoided as much as possible because documentation consisting mainly of abbreviations may not accurately communicate the patient's care. If abbreviations are used, they should be used sparingly.

Abbreviations   Medical documentation traditionally has demonstrated an overuse of abbreviations. Each health discipline has a long list of abbreviations for its unique terminology. Individual clinical facilities also have their lists of acceptable abbreviations, but the lists may differ somewhat from facility to facility. Some abbreviations may be commonly used within a facility, community, or region. However, these same abbreviations may never be used in other facilities or areas or they may be used with different definitions. Table 4–1 lists the medical terms that use the abbreviation *PT* or *PTA*. Davis, in *Medical Abbreviations: 10,000 Conveniences at the Expense of Communication and Safety,*[4] writes

> Abbreviations are sometimes not understood or are interpreted incorrectly. Their use may lengthen the time needed to train individuals in the health fields, at times delay the patient's care and occasionally result in patient harm (p 1).

Davis offers the following example of how the patient's care may be delayed because of the misinterpretation of the abbreviation *PT*.

> The order for PT, intended to signify a lab test order for prothrombin time, resulted in the ordering of a physical therapy consultation (p 1).

Table 4–1 ➤ LIST OF MEDICAL TERMS ABBREVIATED AS PT OR PTA	
PT	**PTA**
Cisplatin	Percutaneous transluminal angioplasty
Parathormone	Physical therapy (sic) assistant*
Parathyroid	Plasma thromboplastin antecedent
Paroxysmal tachycardia	Post traumatic amnesia
Patient	Pretreatment anxiety
Phenytoin	Prior to admission
Phototoxicity	Pure-tone average
Physical therapy	
Pine tar	
Pint	
Posterior tibial	
Preterm	
Prothrombin time	

*Davis uses the term *physical therapy assistant*, which is incorrect. This is a common mistake. Physical therapy personnel must promote the use of the correct term, *physical therapist assistant.*

From Davis, NM: Medical Abbreviations: 10,000 Conveniences at the Expense of Communications and Safety, ed. 7. Neil M Davis Associates, Huntingdon Valley, PA, 1995, pp 176–177.

It cannot be assumed that the reader will take the time to look up the meaning of each unfamiliar abbreviation. For example, an insurance representative who does not understand the abbreviations may deny payment for the patient's care. The use of abbreviations also potentially increases the patient's risk for inappropriate or even dangerous treatment because an abbreviation was misinterpreted. For example, the PTA would make a serious mistake if the abbreviation TWB was interpreted as total weight bearing instead of touch weight bearing for a patient with a recent hip fracture!

Although risky, abbreviations are being used in documentation. Therefore, the student PTA needs to understand the definitions or abbreviations used in physical therapy and know where to find the definitions of other abbreviations. Abbreviations have been used in examples and practice exercises in this text. A list of those abbreviations with their definitions is located in Appendix A. Medical terminology and physical therapy documentation texts are additional resources for abbreviation lists.

Clarity   The meaning of what is written must be immediately clear to the reader. Use words to paint a picture of the patient's functioning and condition. The description should allow the reader to "see" the patient accurately in the mind's eye (e.g., "In sitting position, client grasps pant leg to lift and place L lower leg on R knee to reach L shoe."). See Chapter 6 for instructions on how to describe a patient's functioning.

If the information is handwritten, it must be legible. Information that is difficult to read may be interpreted incorrectly, creating the potential for the provision of unsafe or inappropriate treatment. In addition, payment for treatment may be denied if the insurance representative finds the handwriting too difficult to read. To avoid the problem of poor handwriting, many facilities require that all documentation information be dictated and typed by a medical transcriptionist (information about dictating techniques are in Appendix C). Other facilities have computers with documentation software designed for physical therapy evaluations and notes.

Punctuation, grammar, and spelling must be correct. This demonstrates attention to detail and implies quality work. Spelling errors may suggest carelessness, possibly implying errors in patient care.

Date and Signature   Documentation must be signed with the caregiver's legal signature followed by the abbreviation for his or her professional title (e.g., Sally M. Smith, PTA. Lic. #123). Progress notes written by PTAs do not need to be cosigned by a PT. However, some facilities require that either all notes or certain periodic notes written by the PTA be cosigned by the supervising PT, depending on the facility's interpretation of the criteria set by the insurance company and the state's physical therapy practice act (e.g., Sally M. Smith, PTA/Jane Doe, PT). Notes written by students must be cosigned by the supervising PT or PTA (e.g., Joe Citizen, SPTA/Jane Doe, PTA, Lic. #456).

The APTA is recommending that PTs and PTAs include their license or registration number after their title in all documentation[1] to distinguish themselves from other health-care providers, such as chiropractors, athletic trainers, and massage therapists, who may perform similar treatment measures (e.g., hot packs, whirlpool, ultrasound, and massage). Audits are performed on medical records to determine whether a modality is being overused or used effectively. Adding the license number identifies that the modality was administered by a physical therapy provider.

Every note must be dated, and the date should be easily visible. Usually the date is located in the left margin at the beginning of the note. Figure 4–3 depicts a progress note properly dated and signed.

Use of Black Ink   Use of black ink is a common guideline but subject to change. Black ink traditionally had been used because it copied more clearly than other ink colors. Technology of copying machines has progressed so that other ink colors now copy clearly and print as black in a copy. Some lawyers are now having legal documents signed in blue ink to distinguish the original from the copy. Other colors such as green, mauve, or taupe may copy well but are inappropriate for a medical record. The PTA should follow the facility's procedure.

> 5-14-00 **Dx:** Multiple sclerosis.
> **PT Dx:** Ataxia of lower extremities.
> Patient stated she fell yesterday when attempting to step up onto a curb; second time this week she has fallen. Bruise on left lower leg observed. Patient attempted to step up onto stool and stubbed toe. Coordination exercises performed with emphasis on foot lifting and placement. Home program provided (see written program in chart). Following exercise session, patient accurately placed foot on stool and stepped up independently. Patient is able to control foot placement with visual cues and concentration. Patient to return on 5-21-00 for follow-up. Check on home exercise program and coordination progress per PT plan.
>
> Sue Smith, PTA

Figure 4–3 A progress note properly dated and signed.

No Opportunities for Changing or Falsifying Information

In every case, it should be difficult for someone to change or alter the written note. To ensure that no opportunities exist for changing or falsifying the information, follow these guidelines:

- *Do not use erasable pens.*
- *Do not erase errors.* Draw a line through the mistake, and date and initial directly above the error (e.g., patient ambulated with 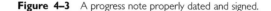 ~~crutches~~ standard walker).
- *Do not leave empty lines or spaces.* Empty spaces provide the opportunity for someone to add or change information, thus falsifying the record. Draw a horizontal line through empty spaces.

Timeliness

Document as soon as possible after seeing the patient, while the information is fresh in your mind. A progress note written immediately after the patient treatment session is the most accurate note. However, it is more likely that the PTA may move from one patient to the next and treat a full day's schedule of patients before being able to document. Carry a small notebook to take notes while treating the patient so that each patient's progress note will be accurate and thorough.

Treatments that are provided twice a day may be documented by placing AM or PM after the date (12-4-00 AM) (12-4-00 PM). This allows another health-care provider, such as the OT, nurse, or speech pathologist, to document in the progress note section of the chart between the physical therapy AM and PM notes, thus illustrating the continuum of care throughout the day. An addendum is made when information is added to a note that has already been written and signed. To add more information later, date the new entry and state "addendum to physical therapy note dated _____." Refer to Figure 4–2 as an example of a progress note that follows legal guidelines.

S U M M A R Y

The PTA writes the progress note to provide proof that the physical therapy treatment plan is being carried out. It is a record of the patient's progress and the effectiveness of the interventions. The progress note may be written in various formats but it is commonly written in narrative paragraph or SOAP outline forms. It is part of a legal record written in accordance with guidelines for legal documentation.

R E F E R E N C E S

1. American Physical Therapy Association: Guidelines for Physical Therapy Documentation. APTA, Alexandria, VA, 1998.
2. Somerness, W: Work Hardening, Specialties in Occupational Medicine. Notes from workshop presentation, August 1986, Superior, Wisconsin.
3. Kettenbach, G: Writing SOAP Notes. FA Davis, Philadelphia, 1995, p 8.
4. Davis, NM: Medical Abbreviations: 10,000 Conveniences at the Expense of Communication and Safety, ed 7. Neil M Davis Associates, Huntingdon Valley, PA, 1995, p 1.

► REVIEW EXERCISES

1. Discuss the importance of the progress note to the medical record, the frequency of writing, and who writes it.

2. List three examples of forms for writing the progress note.

3. List the guidelines for writing in a legal record. Explain the purpose of each guideline.

4. Discuss why the use of abbreviations is not recommended.

5. Explain why APTA recommends that PTs and PTAs include their license numbers when signing physical therapy documentation.

Practice Exercise 1 ➤   *You are reading your new patient's chart and you see the progress note written with so many abbreviations that you are not sure you really understand it. Rewrite the note so it is still as brief as possible, but any reader would understand it. Follow this hospital's SOAP documentation style. Follow guidelines for documenting in a legal record. Use Appendix A to find the definitions for the abbreviations.*

9-17-00   **Dx:** L TKA.

_____

PT Dx: Unable to ambulate ① LLE weakness, PWB allowed.

_____

S: Pt. states he slept "poorly" last two noc. Pt. reported min. c/o pain w/ex. during tx session.

O: Pt. transferred OOB R supine to sit w/mod A ×1. Sat ×5 min w/c/o dizziness. Gt. Trng. w/fw/w PWB L flat surface ×30 ft mod A ×1 ×2 w/5 min rest. Pt. Ret. to bed for ther. Ex. to LLE of quad set 10 reps 5 sec hold w/strong contraction. SLR ×10 reps w/ER to 10° lag. AROM L knee 10–50°, PROM 0–60°.

A: ↑ROM, ↑distance. Pt. making gains even though N/A to sleep well. Pt. expected to achieve STG of ↑ROM, ↑str., and min. A gtP: Cont. w/gt. Trng. & ther. ex. Begin stair amb. PM 9/18/00.

—J. T., PTA

_____

_____

_____

_____

_____

_____

_____

_____

_____

_____

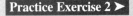

Practice Exercise 2 ➤ *List the* legal guidelines *the PTA did not follow when writing the following progress note (do not attempt to critique the content).*

Dx: Psoriasis both arms
_____

PT Dx: Difficulty sleeping and concentrating due to severe itching.
_____

S: Pt. states R elbow itches alot. States his knees feel stiff, has trouble getting up out of his favorite chair. He likes to sit in his chair with his cat in his lap and they watch the traffic go by.

O: Seen pt. 4 times. Ultraviolet treatment to both arms to dry up the soars. Rash gone from L forearm.

A: Pt. tolerating treatment OK.

P: Continue per PT initial plan.

_____

_____

_____

_____

_____

Practice Exercise 3 ➤ *List the* legal guidelines *the PTA did not follow when writing the following progress note (do not attempt to critique the content).*

11-17-00   **Dx:** L CVA.
_____

   PT Dx: Weakness in RUE & LE with unsafe ambulation and dependent in ADLs.
_____

Pt. states not doing exercises at home. Has not been going out to church or club meetings because she is afraid of falling. Pt. states she has always been active and wishes she could go to her bridge club meetings. She loves to play bridge and misses her bridge club friends the most. They have been friends since they were girls together in grade school. L hand extremely purple! Can't bare wt. on hand due to stiffness in fingers, decreased ROM in all finger joints. Can't push on hand to get up off of floor. Isometrics to shoulder, lots of cheating. ~~AAROM~~ PROM biceps/triceps, shoulder flexion/extension, shoulder internal rotation/external rotation, forarm pronation/supination, shoulder abduction/adduction, wrist flexion/extension, wrist ulnar deviation/radial deviation, 10 reps each in supine position. Independent supine to sit if role to R elbow for support and push with L hand to get up. Pt has difficulty comprehending: and is impatient: and is uncooperative. Will continue treatment 3×wk per PT plan.

—M. Lukan

_____

_____

_____

_____

_____

_____

Practice Exercise 4 ➤ *Rewrite the progress note in Practice Exercise 2 using the correct legal guidelines. This progress note is poorly written, but do not try to improve the content. Correct only errors related to legal guidelines. You will be asked to improve the content of this note in a practice exercise later in the text.*

_____

_____

_____

_____

_____

_____

_____

_____

Practice Exercise 5 ➤ *Rewrite the progress note in Practice Exercise 3 using the correct legal guidelines. This progress note is poorly written, but do not try to improve the content. Correct only errors in legal guidelines. You will be asked to improve the content of this note in a practice exercise later in the text.*

_____

_____

_____

_____

_____

_____

_____

Writing the Content: Subjective Data

LEARNING OBJECTIVES *After studying this chapter, the student will be able to:*
➤ Identify subjective data
➤ Select relevant subjective data to document the patient's physical therapy diagnosis and treatment
➤ Organize subjective data for easy reading and understanding
➤ Demonstrate adherence to the recommended guidelines for documenting subjective data
➤ Use appropriate methods to properly document information about the patient's pain

INTRODUCTION Regardless of the organizational format used, subjective data content in the physical therapy examination and evaluation report and the progress note is typically located at the beginning of or early in the note. For example, it is recorded in the S section of the SOAP outline, in the D section of the DEP format, and in the F section of the FOR. Subjective data content is included in the S (status) section of the PSPG organization. Subjective data are critically important in physical therapy examination and evaluation reports. As part of the continuum of care in progress notes, subjective data provide evidence of treatment effectiveness or progress toward the functional goals.

SUBJECT DATA

Subjective data consists of information that the patient, significant other, or caregiver *tells* the PT and PTA concerning the patient's present condition and treatment.

Relevant Information

One of the key words in the definition for subjective data is *relevant*. Unfortunately, a common mistake seen in progress notes is the inclusion of information that does not relate to the patient's problem, diagnosis, or the treatment session (Fig. 5–1). Confining the subjective information to only that which is relevant is not an easy task. The PTA and the patient will likely have conversations about a variety of subjects. Important information about the patient's problem or diagnosis often slips out during a seemingly unrelated conversation. The PTA must be an alert listener to sort out the relevant information.

Necessary Listening Skills

Effective listening is a skill that is consciously developed with practice. To sort out relevant information, the PTA must be aware that much of the workday is spent listening in a variety of ways. Some listening techniques include:

1. **Analytic** listening for specific kinds of information (e.g., pain, lifestyle, fears)
2. **Directed** listening to a patient's answers to specific questions (e.g., What positions increase frequency or intensity of pain? What does the patient need to be able to do at work?)
3. **Attentive** listening for general information to get the total picture of the patient's situation
4. **Exploratory** listening because of one's own interest in the subject
5. **Appreciative** listening for aesthetic pleasure (e.g., listening to music on headphones while walking during lunch break)
6. **Courteous** listening because it demonstrates respect for the patient
7. **Passive** listening by overhearing (e.g., conversation in the next treatment booth)

Analytic, directed, and attentive listening provides information that may be relevant for subjective data content in the progress note. More relevant information may be revealed when exploratory listening is used.

Examples

The PTA becomes familiar with the patient's medical record by reading the PT's initial examination/evaluation report and the initial evaluation reports of the physician and any other health-care providers treating the patient. During treatment sessions, the PTA should listen for any information that relates to treatment effectiveness and accomplishment of goals and outcomes. The PTA should also report to the PT and document in the progress note any information heard that is not in the record but may be important for effective and quality physical therapy care of the patient.

MEDICAL HISTORY

INITIAL EXAMINATION: Information about the patient's previous medical conditions and treatments are in the medical history section of the medical chart and in the initial examination reports.

11-17-00 **Dx:** L CVA.

PT Dx: Weakness in RUE & LE with unsafe ambulation and dependent in ADLs.

Pt. states not doing exercises at home; has not been going out to church or club meetings because she is afraid of falling. Pt. states she has always been active and wishes she could go to her bridge club meetings. She loves to play bridge and misses her bridge club friends the most. They have been friends since they were girls together in grade school. They just celebrated their 65th year of friendship!

Robert Relevant, SPTA/ Tom Jones, PTA

Figure 5–1 Subjective data section of a progress note containing superfluous information.

PROGRESS NOTE: Listen for any medical history information that was not reported earlier but is relevant to the patient's treatment and record such information in the progress note.

> *Example:* Sue, the PTA, sneezes four times as she escorts Mrs. Smith to the treatment cubicle to prepare for an ultrasound treatment. As she excuses herself to go wash her hands, Sue explains that she is not sick but is allergic to pollen during this time of the year. Mrs. Smith mentions her allergy to a perfume that Sue knows is in the ultrasound gel. As Sue positions Mrs. Smith on the plinth, Mrs. Smith states that she itched for awhile "right where the PT gave my first ultrasound treatment yesterday." Sue makes a mental note to use ultrasound lotion instead of the gel today, to inform the PT, and be sure to document this in the progress note. Figure 5–2 demonstrates how this information is included in the progress note.

ENVIRONMENT: LIFESTYLE, HOME SITUATION, WORK TASKS, SCHOOL NEEDS, AND LEISURE ACTIVITIES

INITIAL EXAMINATION: The PT already will have interviewed the patient to learn about his or her needs at home to help plan treatment goals.

PROGRESS NOTE: Listen for any further information that will influence treatment amd document in the progress note.

> *Example:* Sue knows from reading the medical record that her patient, Harry, has a toilet next to a combination tub and shower with grab bars at home, and that his bathroom is small. Harry had a stroke, and his balance is slightly unsteady. Sue is planning to teach him to slide from the toilet onto the edge of the tub, swing his feet into the tub, then stand for his shower. Today, during his treatment session, Harry's wife comments that her back is aching because she just spent an hour cleaning the shower doors and the track in which the doors slide. "That track is uncomfortable to sit on," thought Sue. "I need to think of a better method for Harry to transfer into his tub."

EMOTIONS OR ATTITUDES

INITIAL EXAMINATION: The PT records the patient's attitude or emotional state presented at the time of the examination.

PROGRESS NOTE: Patient's attitudes can change during the course of treatment, or they might not have presented their true feelings to the PT during the initial examination. The PTA needs to be alert for these changes.

4-19-00 PT Dx: Subdeltoid bursitis with decreased deltoid strength and decreased shoulder ROM interfering with ability to perform work tasks.

S: Pt. reports itching "right where the PT gave my first ultrasound treatment yesterday." Mentioned she is allergic to some perfumes.

O: No skin rash or redness observable in treatment area today. Direct contact US/1 MHz/1.5 w/cm^2 (moderate heat)/5 min/R subdeltoid bursa/sitting/shoulder extended/arm resting on pillow to decrease inflammation. Used ultrasound lotion instead of gel. Gel contains perfume. Pt. correctly performed home exercise program of isometrics for the deltoid, holding for 8 counts (see copy in chart).

Shoulder AROM:	before tx	after tx
flexion	0–55°	0–60°
abduction	0–68°	0–73°

A: Treatment tissue less sensitive to US (1 w/cm^2 yesterday). US effective in reducing inflammation. Pt. beginning to progress toward goal of decreased inflammation, improved shoulder mobility to perform work tasks.

P: Will monitor pt.'s response to the US lotion tomorrow and alert PT of the reaction to the gel. Pt. is scheduled for four more treatments.—Sue Citizen, PTA

Figure 5–2 Adding new relevant subjective information to the medical record through the progress note.

Example: PTA Jim treats his patient Sam, who had a stroke. Yesterday, they worked on balance and stability using the hands-and-knees position and batting a balloon while in sitting position. Today Sam refuses to go to physical therapy. He states that he does not want to play children's games and that if he could just go home, he would be fine. Jim realizes he needs to consult the PT and restructure the treatment sessions to work on balance and stability in activities Sam will want to be doing at home.

GOALS OR FUNCTIONAL OUTCOMES

INITIAL EXAMINATION: Goals or functional outcomes are set by the patient and the PT during the initial evaluation.

PROGRESS NOTE: Goals may need to be modified as the patient and the PTA become better acquainted and the PTA learns more about the patient's needs and desires.

Example: Sam told the PT that he needs to be able to climb only two steps to get into his house; the rest of his house is on one floor. They set a stair-climbing goal: "To be able to climb two steps independently using the railing on the left and be able to ascend and descend a curb independently with no ambulation device." One week later, during a treatment session, Sam is telling Jim about his cabin on a nearby lake and how anxious he is to go to the cabin and go fishing. Sam casually mentions that there are six wooden steps down to the dock. Jim makes a mental note to share this information with the PT and to suggest that the goal be modified.

UNUSUAL EVENTS OR CHIEF COMPLAINTS

INITIAL EXAMINATION: Chief complaints are the patient's symptoms of the disease or dysfunction requiring treatment.

PROGRESS NOTE: During treatment sessions, reports of unusual events may indicate a physiologic change in the patient, or may be evidence of the effectiveness or ineffectiveness of the treatment. Reports may also indicate the patient's compliance and other health conditions encountered during the week.

Example 1: Patient states she did not do her home exercises this week because she had the flu. The PTA will realize that this may be why the patient hasn't progressed this week and that this is relevant information for the subjective data in the progress note.

Example 2: PTA Brenda treats Ray, who has a spinal cord injury. Today she goes to Ray's hospital room to take him to physical therapy. Ray complains he is feeling weak, has chills, and is somewhat light-headed. He doesn't think he can exercise in therapy today. Brenda talks with Ray's nurse and cancels this morning's therapy, writing about Ray's complaints and her conversation with Ray's nurse in the progress notes. Brenda checks on Ray in the afternoon, and he tells her that he has a urinary tract infection and is just now starting the medication. He still feels weak and light-headed. Brenda cancels the afternoon treatment session, describing Ray's complaints in the subjective area of the progress note.

RESPONSE TO TREATMENT

PROGRESS NOTE: Reporting the patient's response documents the effectiveness of treatment and influences future treatment plans.

Example: PTA Brenda treats Robert, who has a mild lumbar disc protrusion and complains of waking up often in the night with tingling in his left leg. During yesterday's treatment session, Brenda showed Robert how to use pillows and a rolled towel to support his spine and maintain proper positioning while sleeping. Today, Robert reports that he awoke only three times last night because of back soreness and didn't have have any tingling in his leg. Brenda makes a mental note to quote Robert in the subjective section of the progress note to provide evidence that her instructions in sleeping positions were effective.

Pt. c/o pain in R shoulder when R arm is hanging down. Lives alone. Pt.'s goal is to play on the college volleyball team this winter. Denies having previous injury or trauma to shoulder. C/o pain when attempting to put on sweater and T-shirts. States he is limited to only a few clothing items he can get into without help. States his shoulder started to ache for no apparent reason. Has been practicing volleyball 6 hr/day for the last 3 weeks.

Figure 5–3 Documentation that randomly presents subjective data, making it difficult to get a clear picture of patient's status.

LEVEL OF FUNCTIONING

INITIAL EXAMINATION: The initial examination describes the patient's functional level at the time of the examination.

PROGRESS NOTE: The patient's description of his or her functional level may help the PTA assess the patient's progress or response to treatment.

> *Example:* PTA Mary is treating Mr. Jones, who had an acute flare-up of osteoarthritis in his hands. His chief complaint during the initial evaluation was inability to dress himself, especially handling buttons and snaps, because of the pain. Today he arrives wearing a sweater, which he said he buttoned without needing to ask for help. This comment may be evidence in the progress note that Mr. Jones has met a goal or outcome.

ORGANIZING SUBJECTIVE DATA

The subjective content in the initial examination report may be more complex and detailed than the subjective information in the progress note. The PT may organize this information into subcategories such as complaints (c/o), history (Hx), environment, and the patient's goals or functional outcomes, behavior, and description of pain. This helps the PT confine the data to only the categories that are relevant. Organizing the content makes it easy to read and to locate information. The example in Figure 5–3 randomly presents subjective data, making it difficult to get a clear picture of the patient's status. In Figure 5–4, the note is rewritten, with the information grouped according to topic.

The PTA needs to document subjective data only if there is an update of the previous information or if there is relevant new information. Usually the content is brief. If the information is about more than one topic category, it should be grouped according to the topics. However, identifying the topic categories may not be necessary. Progress notes may not contain subjective information when relevant information is not provided or when the patient is unable to communicate (e.g., the patient is in a coma) and there is no one else present during the treatment to offer subjective data.

WRITING SUBJECTIVE DATA

Verbs

When documenting subjective data, use verbs to indicate to the reader that the information is being provided by the patient. Commonly used verbs include *states, reports, complains of, expresses, describes,* and *denies.* It is not necessary to repeat the word *patient* (or pt.) After it is used once, it is assumed that all the information in the section was told by the patient, as in the examples in Figure 5–5.

c/o: Pt. c/o pain R shoulder when R arm is hanging down and when attempting to put on sweater and T-shirts. **Hx:** States his shoulder started to ache for no apparent reason. Denies having previous injury or trauma to shoulder. **Home situation:** States lives alone. Has only a few clothing items he can get into without help. **Environment/pt.'s goals:** States he has been practicing volleyball 6 hr/day for the last 3 weeks. Wants to play on the college volleyball team this winter.

Figure 5–4 The documentation in Figure 5–3 rewritten with the information grouped according to topics.

1) Patient states she's allergic to perfume; itched at treatment site following yesterday's treatment. 2) Patient states he is anxious to go fishing; has six steps down to the dock at his cabin. 3) Patient reports he awoke only three times last night; denies having leg tingling and back soreness.

Figure 5–5 Three examples of documentation using the word *patient* once.

Patient Quotations Occasionally using direct patient quotations is better than paraphrasing the patient's comments. Quoting will make the intent of the comment or the relevance to the treatment clearer. The following are appropriate situations in which to quote the patient:

1. To illustrate confusion or loss of memory. (*Example:* Pt. often states, "My mother is coming to take me away from here. I want my mother." Pt. is 90 years old.)
2. To illustrate denial. (*Example:* Pt. insists, "I don't need any help at home. I'll be fine once I get home." Pt. is dependent for transfers and ambulation and lives alone.)
3. To illustrate a patient's attitude toward therapy. (*Example:* Pt. states, "I don't want to play children's games. If I could just go home, I would be fine.")
4. To illustrate the patient's use of abusive language. (*Example:* Pt. yelled to therapist, "Keep your hands off my arm! I'm going to kill you!")

Information from Someone Other Than the Patient Relevant information is often provided by the caretaker or significant other. This is especially true for patients with dementia, speech dysfunction, or altered neurologic function, such as coma, and for infants and young children.

When the information is provided by someone other than the patient, begin the subjective information by stating who provided the information. Be sure to state the reason why the patient could not communicate. (*Example:* All of the following information is provided by pt.'s mother. Pt. is in a coma.)

When information is provided by both the patient and another person, specifically note when it is patient-supplied information and when the information is supplied by the other person. (*Example:* Mrs. Jones states she did not have to help her husband button his sweater today. Mr. Jones states that today is the first time he has not had to ask for help since his arthritis flared up.)

Pain Documentation of pain is unique because it often seems like objective data (Fig. 5–6). Also it may seem as though pain is the judgment or opinion of the therapist. Pain is an element of the subjective data content. Pain information is placed in the S (subjective) section of the SOAP-organized progress note.

The patient's pain experience and perception of its intensity vary widely among individuals. Consider the example about dental experiences. Some never need local anesthesia to have a cavity filled, whereas others need Novocain (procaine hydrochlroide), music in headphones, and other distractions.

Pain is difficult to describe in words. Not only can patients experiencing similar levels of pain use different words to describe that pain, but different therapists may impute different meaning to a patient's words. Because the patient is providing the pain description, this information is documented in the subjective section.

1. Patient rates pain a 6 on an ascending scale of 1–10 when climbing stairs.
2. Patient gives her pain a 4 on a pain scale of 1–7 where 1 is no pain and 7 is excruciating pain.
3. Patient reports his pain is 3/10 after massage compared to 6/10 before massage.
4.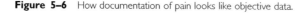
$$\underline{1 \qquad\qquad x \qquad\qquad 1}$$
1 2 3 4 5 6 7 8 9 10

Figure 5–6 How documentation of pain looks like objective data.

There are many words that describe pain. Some of these are grouped below. Check (✔) any words that describe the pain you have these days.

1.
- ☐ Flickering
- ☐ Quivering
- ☐ Pulsing
- ☐ Throbbing
- ☐ Beating
- ☐ Pounding

5.
- ☐ Pinching
- ☐ Pressing
- ☐ Gnawing
- ☐ Cramping
- ☐ Crushing

9.
- ☐ Dull
- ☐ Sore
- ☐ Hurting
- ☐ Aching
- ☐ Heavy

13.
- ☐ Fearful
- ☐ Frightful
- ☐ Terrifying

17.
- ☐ Spreading
- ☐ Radiating
- ☐ Penetrating
- ☐ Piercing

2.
- ☐ Jumping
- ☐ Flashing
- ☐ Shooting

6.
- ☐ Tugging
- ☐ Pulling
- ☐ Wrenching

10.
- ☐ Tender
- ☐ Taut
- ☐ Rasping
- ☐ Splitting

14.
- ☐ Punishing
- ☐ Grueling
- ☐ Cruel
- ☐ Vicious
- ☐ Killing

18.
- ☐ Tight
- ☐ Numb
- ☐ Drawing
- ☐ Squeezing
- ☐ Tearing

3.
- ☐ Pricking
- ☐ Boring
- ☐ Drilling
- ☐ Stabbing

7.
- ☐ Hot
- ☐ Burning
- ☐ Scalding
- ☐ Searing

11.
- ☐ Tiring
- ☐ Exhausting

15.
- ☐ Wretched
- ☐ Blinding

19.
- ☐ Cool
- ☐ Cold
- ☐ Freezing

4.
- ☐ Sharp
- ☐ Cutting
- ☐ Lacerating

8.
- ☐ Tingling
- ☐ Itchy
- ☐ Smarting
- ☐ Stinging

12.
- ☐ Sickening
- ☐ Suffocating

16.
- ☐ Annoying
- ☐ Troublesome
- ☐ Miserable
- ☐ Intense
- ☐ Unbearable

20.
- ☐ Nagging
- ☐ Nauseating
- ☐ Agonizing
- ☐ Dreadful
- ☐ Torturing

Figure 5–7   An example of a checklist pain profile. (Adapted from the McGill Pain Questionnaire.)

Each facility has its own procedure for documenting pain. Typically this information is documented in the pain profile. Several types of pain profiles are commonly used, including pain scales, checklists, and body drawings. Regardless of the pain profile or technique used for documenting the pain, consistency in each note is essential. Inconsistent documentation hinders a determination of treatment effectiveness. Information on a pain scale cannot be compared with information on a body drawing. Changes in the pain profile can be identified by comparing the initial profile with the pain reports throughout the treatment sessions.

Consistent pain documentation provides a clear picture or measurement of treatment effectiveness and helps ensure reimbursement by third-party payers. It is important to understand that pain profiles provide an *objective* method for documenting pain, but the profile is documented in the *subjective* section of the progress note. Students often make the mistake of documenting pain in the objective section.

Pain Scale   Facilities often use a pain profile based on a numbered scale, usually from 0–10 or 1–7 with 0 or 1 designating no pain and 7 or 10 denoting the worst pain imaginable. The patient rates the pain as a number on the scale. This information is recorded in the subjective section (see Fig. 5–6). The scale should be described in the note (e.g., "0 = no pain, 10 = worst pain imaginable"; "1 = no pain, 7 = excruciating"; "on an ascending scale of 0–10.") The pain rating may be documented as 5/10 or 3/7 if the definition of the scale has been described earlier in the record or chart.

Checklist   Another method of documenting pain is a checklist of words describing pain. The patient checks the words that describe his pain. This checklist is inserted in the medical chart, and a note in the subjective section of the progress note instructs the reader to refer to the checklist. Figure 5–7 is an example of a checklist pain profile.

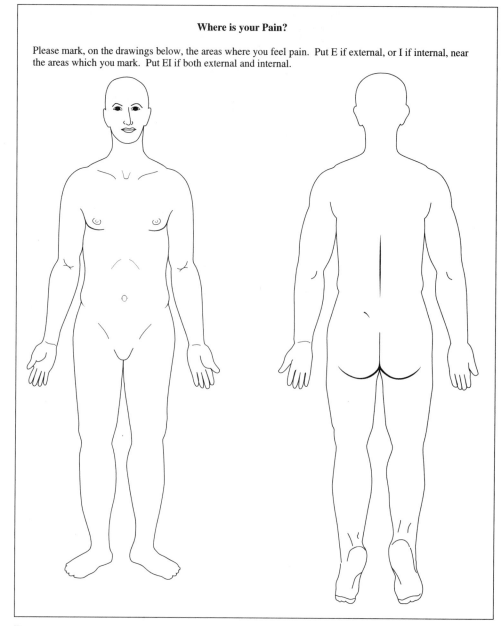

Where is your Pain?

Please mark, on the drawings below, the areas where you feel pain. Put E if external, or I if internal, near the areas which you mark. Put EI if both external and internal.

Figure 5–8   An example of a body-drawing pain profile.

Body Drawing   An outline drawing of the body may be used for the patient to mark the location of the pain. Symbols or colors are used to indicate the type and intensity of the pain at each location. This form is then inserted in the medical chart for pain documentation. Figure 5–8 is an example of a body drawing pain profile.

S U M M A R Y   Information told to the PT or PTA by the patient, significant other, or other caregiver is documented as subjective data in the progress note. The information must be relevant to the patient's treatment and/or physical therapy diagnosis. The PT and PTA use different types of listening to identify relevant information. The information can be paraphrased or quoted verbatim in the progress note. Including subjective information in the progress note when none was provided or when the patient repeated information that had already been documented in previous notes is not necessary. Although appearing more like objective data, comments regarding pain and structured pain profiles are documented with the subjective data.

➤ REVIEW EXERCISES

1. Define subjective data.

2. Discuss the type of subjective data relevant to the patient that should be included in the progress note.

3. Describe the organization of subjective data.

4. Describe the guidelines for writing the subjective data content.

5. Explain why information about pain is subjective data.

6. Discuss two mistakes students often make when writing subjective data.

IDENTIFYING THE PHYSICAL THERAPY PROBLEM AND SUBJECTIVE DATA STATEMENTS

Write "Pr" next to statements that describe the physical therapy problem or diagnosis, and "SD" next to statements that fit the subjective data category.

_____ Pt. states she has a clear understanding of her disease and her prognosis.

_____ Pt. expresses surprise that the ice massage relaxed her muscle spasm.

_____ Muscle spasms L lumbar paraspinals with sitting tolerance limited to 10 min.

_____ Pt. describes tingling pain down back of R leg to heel.

_____ Dependent in ADLs because of flaccid paralysis in R upper and lower extremities.

_____ Sue states her L ear hurts.

_____ Unable to reach behind back because of limited ROM in R shoulder int. rot.

_____ Reports he must be able to return to work as a welder.

_____ Patient states the doctor told her she had a laceration of R vastus medialis.

_____ Paraplegic 2° SCI T12 and dependent in wheelchair transfers.

_____ States Hx of RA since 1980.

_____ Pt. denies pain c̄ cough.

_____ States injury occurred December 31, 1999.

_____ SPTA c/o he has to sit for 2 hours in the PTA lectures.

_____ Grip strength weakness and inability to turn doorknobs to open doors because of carpal tunnel syndrome.

_____ Describes his pain as "burning."

_____ Unable to sit because of decubitus over sacrum.

_____ Unable to feed self because of limited elbow flexion.

_____ Pt. rates her pain a 4 on an ascending scale of 1–10.

_____ States able to sit through a 2-hour movie last night.

1. Identify the statements in Practice Exercise 1 to which you answered "Pr." *Underline* the impairment and *circle* the functional limitation.

2. *Underline* the verb in the statements that clued you to identify the statements as "SD."

3. List the medical diagnoses you can find in the statements.

_____

_____

_____

_____

_____

Practice Exercise 3 ➤

You are treating Nancy, who has been diagnosed as having a mild disc protrusion at L4,5 with spasms in the right lumbar paraspinal muscles. You read in the PT initial examination/evaluation that she reported pain in right low back and buttock areas, and you see the areas marked on a body drawing. The spasms and pain have interfered with Nancy's ability to sit; she is unable to tolerate sitting longer than 15 minutes and unable to sleep more than 2 hours at a time. She also reports having difficulty with bathing and dressing activities. Nancy works as a nursing assistant at the local hospital and has been unable to perform her job tasks. The desired functional outcomes for Nancy are to be able to sit 30 minutes, sleep 5 hours, achieve independence in bathing and dressing, and return to her work as a nursing assistant. The treatment plan and objectives are to include massage to the lumbar paraspinal muscles to relax the spasms, static pelvic traction for 10 minutes to encourage receding of the disc protrusion and stretching and relaxing the lumbar paraspinal muscles, patient education in a home exercise program for lumbar extension and control of the disc protrusion, and instructions on posture and body mechanics for correct and safe sitting, sleeping, bathing, dressing, and performance of work tasks. You have written this progress note:

6-3-00:   **Dx:** Disc protrusion L4,5.

_____

PT Dx: -Muscle spasms lumbar paraspinals with limited sitting, sleeping tolerance, difficulty with ADLs, and unable to perform work tasks.

_____

Patient states she was able to sit through 30 minutes of *The Young and The Restless* soap opera yesterday. Rates her pain a 5 on an ascending scale of 1–10. Patient has received 4 treatment sessions. Decrease in muscle tone palpable after 10-minute massage to right lumbar paraspinal muscles, prone position over one thin pillow. Unable to tolerate lying propped on elbows because of pain before traction, able to lie propped on elbows 5 minutes following 10 minutes, prone, static pelvic traction, 70 pounds. No pain in buttock area. Correctly performed lumbar extension exercises 1, 2, and 3 of home exercise program (see copy in chart) and observed consistently using correct sitting posture with lumbar roll. Patient required frequent verbal cueing for correct body mechanics while performing 10 repetitions (3 reps in initial eval.) of circuit of job simulation activities consisting of bed making, rolling, and moving 30-pound (10-pound in initial eval.) dummy "patient" in bed, pivot transferring the dummy, and wheelchair handling. She did 10 back arches between each task without reminders. Patient has reached 30-minute sitting tolerance outcome, is independent with home exercise program, and compliant with techniques for controlling the protrusion. Progress toward outcome of return to work is 60% with more consistent use of correct body mechanics and ability to lift 50-pound dummy required. Patient to continue treatment sessions 3×/week for 2 more weeks per PT's initial plan. Will notify PT that interim evaluation is scheduled for 6-7-00.

—Sue Smith, PTA, Lic. #0003

Describe what you have done wrong in writing this note and rewrite it correctly.

_____

_____

_____

_____

_____

_____

_____

_____

_____

_____

_____

_____

_____

Practice Exercise 4 ➤ *Place "Yes" next to relevant subjective data statements and "No" next to those that do not seem relevant.*

_____ 1. Client stated her dog was hit by a car last night and she felt too depressed today to do her exercises.

_____ 2. Client reported he progressed his exercises to 50 push-ups yesterday.

_____ 3. Patient's daughter stated she traveled from Iowa, where it has been raining for 2 weeks.

_____ 4. Patient states he does not like the hospital food and is hungry for some Dairy Queen.

_____ 5. Patient rates her pain a 4 on an ascending scale of 1–7.

_____ 6. Patient states she is now able to reach the second shelf of her kitchen cupboard to reach for a glass.

_____ 7. Patient reports he had this same tingling discomfort in his right foot 3 years ago.

_____ 8. Client reports experiencing an aching in his "elbow bone" after the ultrasound treatment yesterday.

_____ 9. Patient says she has 10 grandchildren and 4 great grandchildren.

_____ 10. Client states she forgot to tell the PT that she loves to bowl.

_____ 11. Client reports that *ER* is his favorite TV program.

_____ 12. Client reports he sat in his fishing boat 3 hours and caught a 7-pound Northern Pike this weekend.

_____ 13. Client states he played golf yesterday for the first time since his back injury.

_____ 14. Client states he shot a 56 in golf.

_____ 15. Client states she cannot turn her head to look over her shoulder to back the car out of the garage.

_____ 16. Patient's mother wants to know when her son will come out of the coma.

_____ 17. Client reports he wishes he had not been drinking beer the night of his accident.

_____ 18. Patient describes his flight of stairs with 10 steps, a landing, then 5 more steps and the railing on the right when going up.

_____ 19. Client wishes it would rain, as her prize roses are dying.

_____ 20. Patient states, "I'm going to Macy's to shop and have lunch today." (Patient is 89 years old and is a resident in a long-term care facility in a small town in Ohio. She has been placed on some new medication.)

Writing the Content: Objective Data

LEARNING OBJECTIVES

After studying this chapter, the student will be able to:

➤ Identify objective data
➤ Organize objective data for easy reading and understanding
➤ Demonstrate adherence to recommended guidelines for documenting objective data
➤ Document the patient's functional abilities to provide the reader with a picture of patient functioning
➤ Document interventions so they are reproducible by another PTA or a PT
➤ Document objective data consistent with the data in the PT's initial examination
➤ Identify common mistakes students typically make when documenting objective data

INTRODUCTION

The objective data in the PT's examination report and the PTA's progress note are included with or immediately after the subjective data. These data make up the content of the O (objective) section of the SOAP outline, are included in the data section of the DEP note, are part of the status information in the PSPG-organized note, and are the physical therapy assessment information in the FOR.

The reader of the objective data in the PTA's progress note should be able to form a mental picture of the patient, interventions performed, the patient's response to the interventions, and the patient's functioning before and after the interventions. The PTA should write the objective data so the words paint a picture of the patient and the treatment session. The reader should also be able to clearly understand that the interventions provided during the treatment session require the skills of a physical therapy trained provider (PT or PTA).

OBJECTIVE DATA   Objective data include any information that can be reproduced or observed by someone else with the same training (i.e., another PT or PTA). When written, objective data provide the reader not trained in physical therapy with an understanding of the treatment session and sufficient information to determine whether or not the patient is benefiting from physical therapy. The PTA writes the objective section with two audiences in mind: (1) another PTA (e.g., a replacement PTA in the event you are unable to report to work); and (2) a reader untrained in physical therapy (e.g., an insurance representative, lawyer, quality assurance committee member, physician, or other health-care provider) who is determining the effectiveness of the treatment session.

ORGANIZING OBJECTIVE DATA   Five general topics are appropriate for objective data in the progress note:

1. The results of measurements and tests
2. A description of the patient's function
3. A description of the interventions provided
4. The PTA's objective observations of the patient
5. A record of the number of treatment sessions provided

The information in the objective section of the progress note is organized to flow from one topic to the next, thus making the information easy to read. Similar information should be grouped together. For example, intervention descriptions, results of measurements and tests, and descriptions of the patient's functioning should be organized into three distinct groups.

WRITING OBJECTIVE DATA   The objective data in the initial examination consist of information relevant to the patient's chief complaint and the reason the patient is seeking physical therapy care. These data form the basis for designing the treatment outcomes, goals, and plan. The objective data must consist of measurable, reproducible information so the efficacy of physical therapy treatment procedures can be determined through research of the progress note. When appropriate, the PTA should relate the progress note objective data to the same information in the initial examination or previous notes for comparison. Some objective data can be charted or graphed to provide a quick picture of progress.

Results of Measurements and Tests   All activities or areas specifically mentioned in the initial examination and the outcome and goals from the evaluation should be reassessed and recorded in the progress notes and in the interim and discharge evaluation reports. The PTA determines the patient's progress by re-administering the measurements and tests performed in the initial examination that the PTA is trained to perform. These results are then compared with the results in either the initial examination or in previous progress notes if the patient has been receiving physical therapy for a long period of time. For the comparison to be valid, the retest or measurement must follow the same procedures and techniques that were used when the initial examination was performed. The documentation of the results must also be consistent. For example, if the measurements were in centimeters in the initial examination, they should continue to be documented in centimeters.

The documentation of results may be in the form of either a comment referring the reader to previous results (e.g., "See distance walked in note dated 8-2-00") or an actual written comparison with the results of the previous measurements or tests. Consider the following example.

Example: PTA Sam is treating Mr. Wilson with compression pump therapy to decrease edema in the L ankle. Measurements of the circumference of Mr. Wilson's L ankle were taken in the initial examination (on 8-10-00) to determine the extent of the edema. Today, after 5 treatments, Sam remeasures the circumference of the ankle and compares his results with the initial examination measurements to prove that the edema has decreased and the compression pump intervention is effective.

Sam could record the measurements in a table format in the objective section for easy comparison. Figure 6–1 illustrates measurements presented in table form.

	8-10-00	8-15-00
Center L lat. malleolus	6"	4"
1" inferior to center L lat. malleolus	5.5"	3"
1" superior to center L lat. malleolus	6"	4"
All measurements taken along the superior edge of the marks.		

Figure 6–1   Documentation of measurements in a table form.

In this example, the reader can easily compare results and see that the edema has decreased and the patient is benefiting from the compression pump intervention. Another PTA could follow the directions and duplicate the measurement procedure. Other measurements and tests performed by PTAs, with guidelines for documenting the results, are described in Box 6–1.

▲

● **Box 6–1**   OTHER MEASUREMENTS AND TESTS PERFORMED BY PTAs
WITH GUIDELINES FOR DOCUMENTING THE RESULTS

Guidelines
All measurements and tests must be performed and documented in the same manner as they were performed and documented in the PT initial evaluation. The documentation should include, when applicable:
1. Exactly what is being measured or tested, and on which side.
2. If a motion is being tested, is it passive or active?
3. The position of the patient.
4. The starting and ending points, the boundaries, and the measurement points above and below the starting point.
5. The same scale (e.g. inches, centimeters, degrees) that was used in the initial examination.

Measurements
Tape measurements:
• Girth or circumference
• Leg length
• Wound size
• Step and stride lengths
• Neck and trunk range of motion
Goniometry of all joints

Tests
Manual muscle test of muscle groups
Gross sensory testing

Vital Signs
Heart rate
Respiratory rate
Blood pressure

*Standardized Functional Tests**
Functional Independence Measure
Barthel Assessment
Tinetti Balance
Peabody Developmental Motor Scales
Duke Mobility Status
Posture

---

*These are examples of many tests available.

Description of the Patient's Function

The PTA documents improvement by describing the patient's function.

For example, at the initial examination, Mr. Wilson could not fit his L foot into his running shoe because of the edema in the L foot and ankle. Today, he was able to get his L foot into the shoe with the help of a shoehorn. The next day another PTA could duplicate the assessment by watching Mr. Wilson use a shoehorn to put on his left running shoe. This is a good way to document intervention plan effectiveness because it paints a picture of the patient and describes clearly how the physical therapy interventions are improving the patient's ability to function in his environment. The functional activities must be those specifically mentioned in the goals or functional outcomes in the initial evaluation.

When a comparison of the data shows that the patient's functional status has not changed, be sure all methods for measuring change have been used. For example, a patient may continue to need the assistance of one person for ambulation, but the time it takes the patient to walk from bed to bathroom has decreased. Include the following information when describing the patient's function:

1. The function (e.g., ambulation, transferring, stair climbing, lifting, sweeping, sitting, standing, moving from sit to stand or stand to sit)
2. Description of the quality of the movement when performing the function (e.g., even weight bearing, smooth movement, correct body mechanics, speed)
3. Level of assistance needed (i.e., ranging from independence, verbal reminders; tactile guidance; supervision; standby assist or contact guard assist; minimal, moderate, maximal assist; to dependent)
4. Purpose of the assistance (e.g., verbal cueing for gait pattern, for recovery of loss of balance, for added strength, to monitor weight bearing, to guide walker)
5. Description of equipment needed (e.g., ambulation aids, orthotics, supports, railings, wheelchair, assistive devices)
6. Distances, heights, lengths, times, weights (e.g., 300 ft, 10 meters, 6 min, top shelf of standard-height kitchen cabinet, floor to table, 20 lb)
7. Environmental conditions (e.g., level surface, carpeting, dim light, outside, ramps, low seat)
8. Cognitive status and any complicating factors (patient understanding, ability to follow directions, fainting easily, blood pressure needing monitoring)

Standardized Functional Assessments

For assessing functional abilities, many tools with set protocols and procedures, clear instructions, and methods for rating or scoring the level of function are available. Examples of these tests are the Tinetti Balance Test, Peabody Developmental Motor Scales, Barthel Assessment, Duke Mobility Skills, and Functional Independence Measure. If a standardized assessment tool is used in the initial examination, the PTA, when trained in the use of the tool, can reassess the patient's functional abilities and refer the reader of the progress note to the copy of the completed assessment form in the chart. The assessment tool describes the function and changes in the rating score as evidence of improvement in functional abilities and progress toward the functional outcome identified in the initial evaluation.

Description of the Interventions Provided

The objective data may include information about the treatment procedures that the patient received. Facilities differ in how intervention details are recorded. The interventions may be described in the progress note, recorded on a flow chart, or described on a separate form elsewhere in the chart. In addition, this information may be a combination of narrative progress notes with a checklist type chart. Besides being recorded in the medical record, the interventions are often detailed on a cardex located in the physical therapy department. The PTA should follow the procedures of the facility.

Intervention details must be complete and thorough so the intervention can be duplicated by another PT or PTA. The following information should be included for the intervention description to be reproducible.

1. Identification of the modality, exercise, or activity
2. Dosage, number of repetitions, and distance
3. Identification of the exact piece of equipment, when applicable
4. Settings of dials or programs on equipment
5. Target tissue or treatment area
6. Purpose of the treatment
7. Patient positioning
8. Duration, frequency, and rest breaks
9. Other information that the therapist needs to be aware of that is outside standard procedure or protocol. For example, a cane is adjusted higher than the height determined by standard procedure because the increased height provided greater assistance to the patient for ambulation.
10. Anything that is unique to the treatment of that particular patient; for example, complicating factors, such as taking the patient's pulse rate every 5 minutes.

Appendix B provides guidelines for documenting specific direct interventions.

The intervention description should include or be combined with a description of the patient's response to the intervention. For example: Decreased muscle spasm (decreased tone) was palpable following ice massage, to numbing response (7 min), L paraspinal mms, L3–5, with pt. prone over one pillow.

The details of the intervention can also be included to describe function. For example: Following instructions, pt. safely ambulated with axillary crutches, no wt. bearing on L, from bed to dining room (50 ft) on tiled level surface with standby assist for support for loss of balance recovery 2×.

In these two examples, a reader untrained in physical therapy can visualize the patient's performance, and another PTA could duplicate the interventions the following day.

A copy of any written instructions or information provided to the patient as part of the treatment session should be placed in the medical record. Frequently the PTA will give the patient or a caregiver written instructions for exercises or activities that were taught during the treatment session. This is noted in the objective data, and the reader is informed that a copy is in the chart. When the reader can reproduce the intervention by following the written instructions on the handout, it is not necessary to describe the exercises in the progress note. Figure 6–2 illustrates objective documentation of a treatment session that includes instructing the patient in a home exercise program. In the objective data section, any equipment that was given, lent, or sold to the patient should be mentioned.

PTA's Objective Patient Observations   A description of what the PTA sees or feels (visual and tactile observations) constitutes objective data if it is an observation that another PT or PTA would also make because they have the same training. The observation could be duplicated or confirmed by another PT or PTA. Two examples of objective observations are: (1) reddened skin over a bony area after application of hot packs, such as "a nickel-size, reddened area noted over inferior angle of left scapular after hot pack treatment"; and (2) a description of the patient's gait pattern or how

---

O: Following verbal instructions and demonstrations, pt. accurately performed home exercise program designed to strengthen R hip abductors, extensors, and quadriceps, 5 reps of each ex. today. Pt. provided written instructions, refer to copy in chart.

O: Pt. accurately demonstrated set-up of home cervical polyaxial traction unit; gave self 10-min intermittent traction,15 lb, approximately 5 sec on, 3 sec off, supine. Pt. provided written instructions, see copy in chart.

Figure 6–2 Objective documentation of a treatment session that included instructing the patient in a home exercise program.

the patient walks, such as "client walks with an antalgic gait; trunk held in a slightly forward-leaning posture, minimal arm swing, no pelvic rotation, uneven step length (shorter on right), and shortened stance time on right."

Proof of the Necessity of Skilled Physical Therapy Services

The reader of the progress note must come to the conclusion that the physical therapy services the patient received required the unique skills of physical therapy–trained personnel. With this in mind, the PTA should constantly be mentally asking, "Could someone not trained in physical therapy do what I have just described?" If the instructions presented in this chapter are being followed, the PTA is well on the way to writing the objective data so it describes the need for skilled services. Comparing the objective data in the progress note with the objective data in the initial examination is one way of proving that skilled services are needed.

Careful selection of words also is important. For example, PTs and PTAs do not walk/ambulate or transfer their patients; they *teach* or *train* their patients to ambulate or transfer. Therefore, the intervention described in the progress note should be listed as *gait training* or *transfer training*. The note should describe the patient's response to the training or indicate whether the patient understood the instructions or learned the skill or technique. (e.g., "During gait training, patient ambulated with axillary crutches, NWB on left, needing contact guard assist for security when recovering from occasional loss of balance, 30' on carpeting, 5×, responding to verbal cues for correct posture and proper step-through pattern by needing frequent cueing first 2× and improving to needing one cue 5th ×.") When the patient is taught something, such as exercises, body mechanics, or posture, the note should document that the patient gave a return demonstration of what was taught and whether the demonstration was correct or the patient needed further instructions. Again, the note should use words to "paint a picture" of the patient.

Record of Treatment Sessions

The progress note should keep track of the patient's attendance by recording the number of treatment sessions that have been provided. "Documenting attendance reflects the patient's compliance and participation in rehabilitation."[1] The note should also identify appointments that the patient did not keep and the reason for not attending. When a third-party payer has limited the number of treatment sessions that a patient may receive, the progress note can be a method for tracking the number of sessions for discharge planning. The objective data section can report the number of times the patient has been treated, and the information in the plan section of the note can state how many more treatment sessions are scheduled in the future.

Common Student Mistakes with Objective Data Documentation

The major mistake PTA students make when writing objective data, especially when documenting the interventions provided, is reporting what they did and not how the patient responded or performed; for example, "Instructed pt. in crutch walking, non–wt.-bearing L". This statement refers to what the therapist did. However, it does not give the reader a picture of the patient's performance. The objective section of the progress note is about the *patient*—it should describe the patient's response to the interventions. Examples of progress notes written by students describing what they did are found in Figure 6–3. Figure 6–4 illustrates those notes rewritten to include information about the patient's response.

Another common problem is the tendency to ramble when first learning to document. Organizing the information according to topics prevents rambling. Figure 6–5 is an example of an unorganized objective section of a progress note. Figure 6–6 is the same note, but with the information grouped by topic.

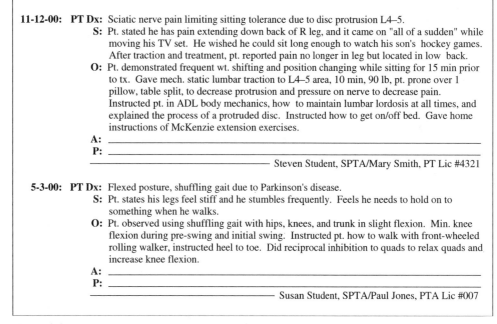

11-12-00: **PT Dx:** Sciatic nerve pain limiting sitting tolerance due to disc protrusion L4–5.

S: Pt. stated he has pain extending down back of R leg, and it came on "all of a sudden" while moving his TV set. He wished he could sit long enough to watch his son's hockey games. After traction and treatment, pt. reported pain no longer in leg but located in low back.

O: Pt. demonstrated frequent wt. shifting and position changing while sitting for 15 min prior to tx. Gave mech. static lumbar traction to L4–5 area, 10 min, 90 lb, pt. prone over 1 pillow, table split, to decrease protrusion and pressure on nerve to decrease pain. Instructed pt. in ADL body mechanics, how to maintain lumbar lordosis at all times, and explained the process of a protruded disc. Instructed how to get on/off bed. Gave home instructions of McKenzie extension exercises.

A: _____

P: _____

——————————————————————— Steven Student, SPTA/Mary Smith, PT Lic #4321

5-3-00: **PT Dx:** Flexed posture, shuffling gait due to Parkinson's disease.

S: Pt. states his legs feel stiff and he stumbles frequently. Feels he needs to hold on to something when he walks.

O: Pt. observed using shuffling gait with hips, knees, and trunk in slight flexion. Min. knee flexion during pre-swing and initial swing. Instructed pt. how to walk with front-wheeled rolling walker, instructed heel to toe. Did reciprocal inhibition to quads to relax quads and increase knee flexion.

A: _____

P: _____

——————————————————————— Susan Student, SPTA/Paul Jones, PTA Lic #007

Figure 6–3 Examples of students' common mistake of writing the objective section of the progress note in terms of what they did.

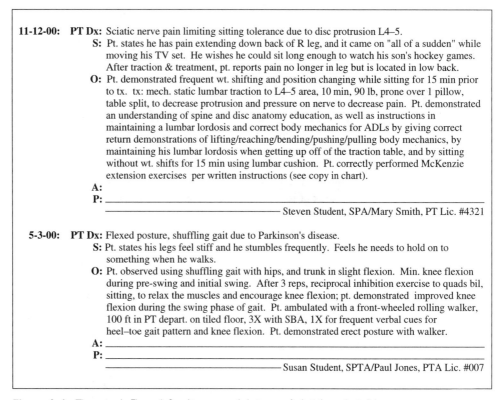

11-12-00: **PT Dx:** Sciatic nerve pain limiting sitting tolerance due to disc protrusion L4–5.

S: Pt. states he has pain extending down back of R leg, and it came on "all of a sudden" while moving his TV set. He wishes he could sit long enough to watch his son's hockey games. After traction & treatment, pt. reports pain no longer in leg but is located in low back.

O: Pt. demonstrated frequent wt. shifting and position changing while sitting for 15 min prior to tx. tx: mech. static lumbar traction to L4–5 area, 10 min, 90 lb, prone over 1 pillow, table split, to decrease protrusion and pressure on nerve to decrease pain. Pt. demonstrated an understanding of spine and disc anatomy education, as well as instructions in maintaining a lumbar lordosis and correct body mechanics for ADLs by giving correct return demonstrations of lifting/reaching/bending/pushing/pulling body mechanics, by maintaining his lumbar lordosis when getting up off of the traction table, and by sitting without wt. shifts for 15 min using lumbar cushion. Pt. correctly performed McKenzie extension exercises per written instructions (see copy in chart).

A:

P: _____

——————————————————————— Steven Student, SPA/Mary Smith, PT. Lic. #4321

5-3-00: **PT Dx:** Flexed posture, shuffling gait due to Parkinson's disease.

S: Pt. states his legs feel stiff and he stumbles frequently. Feels he needs to hold on to something when he walks.

O: Pt. observed using shuffling gait with hips, and trunk in slight flexion. Min. knee flexion during pre-swing and initial swing. After 3 reps, reciprocal inhibition exercise to quads bil, sitting, to relax the muscles and encourage knee flexion; pt. demonstrated improved knee flexion during the swing phase of gait. Pt. ambulated with a front-wheeled rolling walker, 100 ft in PT depart. on tiled floor, 3X with SBA, 1X for frequent verbal cues for heel–toe gait pattern and knee flexion. Pt. demonstrated erect posture with walker.

A: _____

P: _____

——————————————————————— Susan Student, SPTA/Paul Jones, PTA Lic. #007

Figure 6–4 The notes in Figure 6–3 written correctly in terms of what the patient did.

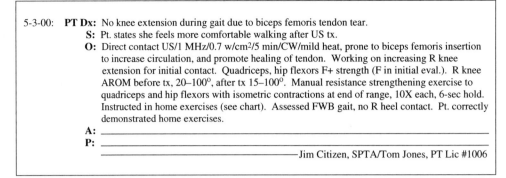

5-3-00: **PT Dx:** No knee extension during gait due to biceps femoris tendon tear.
    S: Pt. states she feels more comfortable walking after US tx.
    O: Direct contact US/1 MHz/0.7 w/cm^2/5 min/CW/mild heat, prone to biceps femoris insertion to increase circulation, and promote healing of tendon. Working on increasing R knee extension for initial contact. Quadriceps, hip flexors F+ strength (F in initial eval.). R knee AROM before tx, 20–100°, after tx 15–100°. Manual resistance strengthening exercise to quadriceps and hip flexors with isometric contractions at end of range, 10X each, 6-sec hold. Instructed in home exercises (see chart). Assessed FWB gait, no R heel contact. Pt. correctly demonstrated home exercises.
    A: _____
    P: _____
              —— Jim Citizen, SPTA/Tom Jones, PT Lic #1006

Figure 6–5   A disorganized objective section of the progress note in which the information rambles.

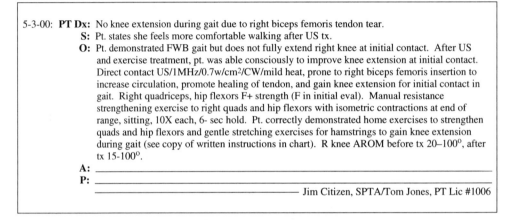

5-3-00: **PT Dx:** No knee extension during gait due to right biceps femoris tendon tear.
    S: Pt. states she feels more comfortable walking after US tx.
    O: Pt. demonstrated FWB gait but does not fully extend right knee at initial contact. After US and exercise treatment, pt. was able consciously to improve knee extension at initial contact. Direct contact US/1MHz/0.7w/cm^2/CW/mild heat, prone to right biceps femoris insertion to increase circulation, promote healing of tendon, and gain knee extension for initial contact in gait. Right quadriceps, hip flexors F+ strength (F in initial eval). Manual resistance strengthening exercise to right quads and hip flexors with isometric contractions at end of range, sitting, 10X each, 6- sec hold. Pt. correctly demonstrated home exercises to strengthen quads and hip flexors and gentle stretching exercises for hamstrings to gain knee extension during gait (see copy of written instructions in chart). R knee AROM before tx 20–100°, after tx 15-100°.
    A: _____
    P: _____
              —— Jim Citizen, SPTA/Tom Jones, PT Lic #1006

Figure 6–6   The note in Figure 6–5 rewritten with the information organized.

SUMMARY   The objective data content of the progress note provides proof of interventions performed, their effectiveness, and the extent of patient improvement, if any. This content must be measurable and reproducible. Objective data content includes intervention details, comparison of results of measurements and tests with previous results, visual and tactile observations made by the PTA, and descriptions of the patient's functional abilities. It should be written so the words paint a picture of the patient and the treatment session and the reader can visualize how the patient is functioning. The objective data content must be relevant to the chief complaint, the goals or functional outcomes, and the reason for the provision of skilled physical therapy services.

REFERENCES   1. Baeten, AM, et al: Documenting Physical Therapy: The Reviewer Perspective. Butterworth-Heinemann, Boston, 1999, p 41.

➤ REVIEW EXERCISES

1. Describe the criteria for information to be considered *objective* data.

2. List the types of information included in the objective data content.

3. Describe how results of tests and measurements are documented.

4. Explain what information should be included when describing the patient's function.

5. Describe what information should be included for the interventions to be reproducible.

6. Describe the two commonest mistakes students make when documenting objective data.

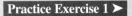

Practice Exercise 1 ➤ **IDENTIFYING THE PROBLEM, SUBJECTIVE DATA, AND OBJECTIVE DATA STATEMENTS**

Write "Pr" next to the problem or PT diagnosis statements, "SD" next to the subjective data statements, and "OD" next to the objective data statements. Answers to numbers 3, 6, 9, 12, 15, and 18 are in the Instructor's Guide, not in this text.

_____ 1. Pt. c/o pain with prolonged sitting.

_____ 2. Decubitus on sacrum measures 3 cm from L outer edge to R outer edge.

_____ 3. Pt. ambulates with ataxic gait, 10 ft max. assist of 2 to prevent fall.

_____ 4. R knee flexion PROM 30–90°.

_____ 5. Ambulates c̄ standard walker, PWB L, bed to bathroom (20 ft), tiled surface, min. assist 1× for balance, verbal cueing for gait pattern.

_____ 6. Pt. states he is fearful of crutch walking.

_____ 7. Limited ROM in L shoulder secondary to fractured greater tubercle of humerus and unable to put on winter coat without help.

_____ 8. c/o itching in scar R knee.

_____ 9. Transfers: supine ↔ sit c̄ min. assist of 1 for strength.

_____ 10. Unable to feed self with L hand because of limited elbow ROM 2° Fx L olecranon process.

_____ 11. AROM WNL bil. LEs.

_____ 12. Pt. demonstrated adequate knee flexion during initial swing c̄ verbal cueing p hamstring exercises.

_____ 13. Dependent in bed mobility due to dislocated R hip.

_____ 14. Expresses concern over lack of progress.

_____ 15. L shoulder flexion PROM 0–100°, lat. rot. PROM 0–40°.

_____ 16. Kathy reports PTA courses are easy.

_____ 17. Pt. pivot transfers, NWB R, bed ↔ w/c, max. assist 2× for strength, balance, NWB cueing.

_____ 18. Pt. rates L knee pain 5/10 when going up stairs.

_____ 19. LUE circumference at 3 cm superior to olecranon process is 12 cm.

_____ 20. BP 125/80 mmHg, pulse 78 BPM, regular, strong.

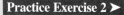

Practice Exercise 2 ➤   *Use the list of statements in Practice Exercise 1 as well as your answers to them.*

1. In the "Pr" statements, underline the impairment and circle the functional limitation.

2. In the "SD" statements, underline the key verb that led you to write "SD."

3. In the "OD" statements, underline the key information that led you to write "OD."

4. List the medical diagnoses you can find in the statements.

_____

_____

_____

_____

_____

_____

_____

Practice Exercise 3 ➤   *Refer to the general documentation guidelines in Box 6–1, and critique each of the following statements that document the results of a test or measurement. Write what is missing or wrong, if anything, in the documentation. The first question is answered for you to illustrate what you are to do.*

1. Left knee flexion PROM 0–63° in sitting position (0–55° in initial exam.).

   There is nothing wrong with this documentation. What is being measured is left knee flex-

   ion; motion is passive; measurements have a starting and ending point; patient position is

   sitting, measurements are consistent with the initial examination.

2. Decubitus over sacrum 3.25 inches from left border to right border, 7 cm in initial exam.

   _____

   _____

   _____

   _____

   _____

3. Hip ROM 75°.

   _____

   _____

   _____

4. Hip abductor strength G- (good minus), 3/5 in initial exam.

_____

_____

_____

5. Left hip hyperextension with anterior pelvic tilt, prone, 20°.

_____

_____

_____

6. Circumference at right olecranon process 4 inches, upper arm 6 inches, lower arm 3 inches.

_____

_____

_____

_____

7. Blood pressure 120/70, pulse 72.

_____

_____

_____

_____

8. Circumference right wrist, supine, UE elevated 45°, 3rd metacarpal head 8 inches, 2 inches superior to 3rd metacarpal head 8 inches, superior edge of ulnar styloid process 7 cm, taken along superior border of marks.

_____

_____

_____

_____

9. Resting respiratory rate 12 breaths per minute relaxed, quiet, sitting position.

_____

_____

_____

_____

10. Left shoulder flexion 100°, abduction 100°, external rotation 60°, internal rotation 40°.

_____

_____

_____

_____

11. Left knee flexion PROM, prone with towel under thigh, 20–110° (30–90° initial exam).

_____

_____

_____

_____

12. Right leg 1 inch longer than left.

_____

_____

_____

_____

13. Trunk forward bend 20%.

_____

_____

_____

_____

14. Trunk side bend greater on right than left.

_____

_____

_____

_____

15. Cervical rotation to right 0–25°, aligned with nose, sitting position, shoulders stabilized.

_____

_____

_____

_____

_____

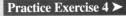 **Practice Exercise 4 ➤** *Refer to documentation guidelines in Box 6–1 and the checklist below taken from the suggestions for documenting interventions in Appendix B, and critique the following statements documenting interventions. Could you reproduce the treatment? If not, what is missing? The first question is answered for you to illustrate what you are to do.*

Type of intervention

Dosage or intensity

Treatment area

Time or duration

Patient position

Frequency

Purpose

1. US/1.5 w/cm2/right shoulder.

   Cannot be reproduced. For the PTA student early in training, the obvious missing information is the time or how long the ultrasound is given, the position of the patient, and the purpose for the ultrasound. The PTA student who has been trained in the theory and application of ultrasound should also recognize that the type of ultrasound is not identified (direct, immersion, continuous, pulsed); the treatment area is not specific enough; and the frequency of the ultrasound (1 MHz or 3 MHz) is not identified. In this case the frequency of treatment, meaning twice a day, daily, every other day, etc., may not be applicable, but the frequency of the ultrasound provided is applicable.

2. Low back massage.

_____

_____

_____

_____

_____

_____

_____

_____

3. Strengthening exercises for quads, hams, and gluts: sets/right/5 sec hold/10 reps each/supine/following 1 hr on knee CPM.

_____

_____

_____

_____

_____

_____

_____

_____

4. Exercises to increase ROM left shoulder.

_____

_____

_____

_____

_____

_____

_____

_____

5. Cervical traction/15 min/14 lb/to stretch muscles.

_____

_____

_____

_____

_____

_____

_____

_____

6. Tilt table/20 min/45°.

_____

_____

_____

_____

_____

_____

_____

_____

7. Home exercise program to increase left knee ROM and strengthen left quads for stair climbing to get to upstairs bathroom (see copy in chart).

_____

_____

_____

_____

_____

_____

_____

_____

8. Phonophoresis/left/subacromial bursa/sitting/to decrease inflammation.

_____

_____

_____

_____

_____

_____

_____

_____

9. High voltage E-stim/motor response/right rhomboids & middle trapezius/to relax spasms.

_____

_____

_____

_____

_____

_____

_____

_____

10. Mechanical pelvic traction/intermittent/30 sec on, 10 sec off/supine (90–90)/90 lb/30 min/to encourage posterior pelvic tilt and stretch lumbar extensor muscles/to decrease lordotic posture.

_____

_____

_____

_____

_____

_____

_____

_____

_____

Practice Exercise 5 ➤

The following are treatment scenarios in which you are the PTA working on functional activities with your patients. Paint a picture of each patient's functioning as if being recorded in the objective data section of your progress note. It is not difficult to paint a picture of the patient's functioning. Just mentally reproduce the treatment session and write the description of the patient performing the activity and how the patient responded to what you are doing. Refer to page 78 for documentation guidelines.

1. You instructed Mrs. Smith, who has severely sprained her right ankle, in crutch walking using a non–weight-bearing gait. Her ankle has been casted, and she is not allowed to bear weight on the right for 3 days. You fitted her with axillary crutches and taught her how to walk 100 ft on tiled and carpeted level surfaces; how to sit down and get up from bed, chair, and toilet; how to climb a flight of stairs with the railing on the right going up; how to manage curbs and two steps without using a railing; and how to get in and out of her car. Mrs. Smith safely ambulated and required only verbal cueing from you to climb the stairs. You gave her written crutch-walking instructions.

_____

_____

_____

_____

_____

_____

_____

_____

2. You supervised Jack practicing his circuit of job-simulation activities using correct body mechanics for 20 minutes, 15 repetitions. Jack has had back surgery (laminectomy L4,5) and is preparing to return to work as a bricklayer. You observed that he consistently maintained his correct lumbar curve when squatting to lift bricks and shifting weight to spread

the mortar. He did need body mechanics reminders when he lifted the wheelbarrow handles and while wheeling the wheelbarrow, especially for turns. He tended to bend from the waist to reach the handles and to twist his trunk when turning the wheelbarrow.

_____

_____

_____

_____

_____

_____

_____

_____

3. You taught Sally, a patient with paraplegia from a spinal cord injury, how to transfer from her wheelchair to the toilet using a sliding board. She required constant instructions and cueing regarding safety precautions, and you needed to help push her across the board. You felt as though you did most of the work. The third time she tried, she was able to slide herself from the chair to the toilet with only a little boost from you. However, when going from the toilet to the chair, it felt as though you and Sally exerted equal effort.

(hint: max. assist = therapist does most of the work; mod. assist = therapist and patient exert about equal effort; min. assist = patient does most of the work)

_____

_____

_____

_____

_____

_____

_____

_____

4. You provided gait training for Mr. Olson to learn to ambulate with a wide-base quad cane in his left hand. He had a stroke and has right upper and lower extremity weakness. You walked with him from his bed into the bathroom, to the bedroom window, out into the hall area in front of his door, and back to his wheelchair next to the bed. He walked this circuit

five times, with a 2-minute rest in the wheelchair between each trip. You needed to hold his gait belt and to help him shift his weight to his right leg. He stumbled three times, but he was able to recover his balance without your help. During the fourth and fifth trips, he was able to shift weight to the right appropriately without your help.

_____

_____

_____

_____

_____

_____

_____

_____

Writing the Content: Diagnoses, Functional Outcomes, Goals, and Treatment Effectiveness

LEARNING OBJECTIVES

After studying this chapter, the student will be able to:

➤ Describe the significance of the subjective and objective data in the progress note
➤ Identify the qualities of a properly written goal
➤ Discuss why the interpretation of the data is the most important portion of the progress note
➤ Explain the topics to be included when the PTA interprets the progress note data
➤ Connect the information in the progress note to the information in the PT's initial evaluation
➤ Write a progress note without making common mistakes

INTRODUCTION

After reviewing subjective and objective data, the informative facts, a person reading the medical record may ask, "What does it mean?" Readers of the record who are not trained in physical therapy (e.g., insurance representatives, lawyers, physicians) may not understand the subjective and objective data unless they are interpreted. The interpretation and significance of the subjective and objective data are reflected in the initial evaluation report, the physical therapy diagnosis, the treatment plan and goals, and the treatment outcomes and effectiveness. These elements of the record support the necessity of the physical therapy medical treatment. The PTA documents the significance of the data in the progress note by describing the patient's response to the treatment plan and the patient's progress toward the accomplishment of the goals. This information is located in the A (assessment) section of the SOAP outline, the E (evaluation) section of the DEP format, and the problems and functional outcome goals portions of the FOR. The information is scattered throughout the PSPG-organized progress note. The physical therapy diagnosis or problem constitutes the first P (problem) section. The rationale for modified treatment plans contained in the second P (plan) section is based on the significance of the data. Discussion about progress toward goals is provided in the G section. For ease of discussion in this chapter, the information will be referred to as *interpretation of the data content*. Interpretation of the data content is more complex in the PT's evaluation reports than in the PTA's progress notes.

INTERPRETATION OF THE DATA CONTENT IN THE EVALUATION

The APTA's *Guidelines for Physical Therapy Documentation* states that the evaluation report should include the physical therapy diagnosis or problem and the goals to be accomplished.[1] By organizing the evaluation information in SOAP format, the PT places this information in the A section. This section contains the PT's interpretation of the signs and symptoms, test results, and observations made during the examination, as well as a conclusion or judgment about the meaning or relevance of the information. The physical therapy diagnoses are based on this interpretation. Desired functional outcomes and anticipated goals are based on the problems. Thus, the subjective and objective information is summarized, and the "what does it mean?" question is answered.

The Physical Therapy Diagnosis/Problem

The first conclusion the PT reaches after evaluating the data is the identification of the physical therapy diagnosis or problem (see Chapter 2).

Outcomes and Goals

The PT and the patient (or a representative of the patient) collaborate to establish the expected functional outcomes and anticipated goals for the physical therapy treatment. The *Guide to Physical Therapist Practice* indicates that *goals* generally address impairments and *outcomes* relate to the patient's functional limitations or reason he or she is receiving therapy.[2]

Expected Functional Outcomes

The expected functional outcome is a broad statement describing the functional abilities necessary for the patient to no longer require physical therapy. *Functional abilities* are the abilities to perform activities or tasks that support the individual's physical, social, and psychological well-being, creating a personal sense of meaningful living.[2] When these abilities are regained, the patient's functional limitations and the disability identified in the physical therapy diagnosis or problem will be eliminated or decreased in severity. This is the criterion for the conclusion of the episode of physical therapy care. The *Guide to Physical Therapist Practice* defines *episode of physical therapy care* as:

> "All physical therapy services that are (1) provided by a physical therapist or under the direction and supervision of a physical therapist, (2) provided in an unbroken sequence, and (3) related to the physical therapy interventions for a given condition or problem ..."[2]

During a patient's episode of care, he or she may transfer to another facility (perhaps more than once) to receive a continuum of physical therapy services. Outcomes may be developed that describe the functional abilities the patient will need to accomplish in order to be discharged from one facility and be transferred to the next. These short-term outcomes are the steps to accomplishing the expected functional outcome. For example, the patient who has undergone total knee-replacement surgery desires to return to independence in walking throughout her home and in the community. This becomes the expected functional outcome for this patient's episode of physical therapy care. The hospital therapy works toward the short-term outcome of independent ambulation with a walker in bedroom, bathroom, and short distances in the hall. When the patient is transferred to a rehabilitation facility, therapy is directed toward the short-term outcome of independent ambulation with an appropriate ambulation aid for longer distances and on carpeting, grass, gravel, stairs, and ramps. When this is accomplished, the patient is discharged and transferred to home where the home health therapist works toward the expected functional outcome for this episode of care, independent ambulation without an ambulation aid in the home and community.

Anticipated Goals

Anticipated goals describe the changes in the impairments necessary for the patient's function to improve. They are the steps for accomplishing the outcomes and thus should relate to the outcomes. For example, goals may describe the desired strength gain, range of motion improvement, and balance improvement needed for the outcome to be accomplished. They may describe the progression of the quality of the movement, the efficiency of the task, and the assist needed to eventually accomplish the functional outcome.

Writing the Functional Outcomes and Goals

Outcomes and goals must be written to include the **action or performance** (e.g., will ambulate), the **measurable criteria** that determine whether a task has been accomplished (e.g., walked from bedroom to kitchen), and a **time period** within which it is expected the outcome or goal will be met (e.g., in 1 week). Measurable criteria are the most important part of the outcome and goal. An action or performance can be measured in a variety of ways. A few examples of measurable criteria are strength grade, degrees of joint motion, scores on standardized test, seconds/minutes, description of the quality of the movement, proper posture/body mechanics, correct techniques, amount of assist needed, assistive equipment needed, and pain rating. When goals address specific impairments, they should also describe how the desired change in the impairment relates to the desired change in the functional limitation. A description of the change in function becomes another method of measuring the accomplishment of the goal. *A description of the change in function becomes the best measurement to ensure third-party reimbursement.* Examples of expected functional outcomes and anticipated goals are given in Figure 7–1. Writing the outcomes and goals in this manner gives the PTA direction for planning treatment sessions that include activities enabling the patient's progression toward the goal, methods for measuring the patient's progress, and standards for determining when to recommend termination of treatment.

Examples of goals relating to the desired change in the impairments and functional limitations include the following:

■ ROM for left shoulder flexion will improve to 0–110 degrees so patient can reach top of head for grooming in 2 weeks.
■ Strength of right gluteus medius will increase to 4/5 so patient will no longer demonstrate a significant trunk shift to the right during stance phase of ambulation in 4 weeks.
■ Amount of edema will decrease so girth measurements of right upper arm will be within 1 inch of left upper arm and patient's right arm will fit into the sleeves of her clothing in 1 week.

In the first goal, the action or performance is improvement in shoulder flexion, the measurable criteria are ROM 0–110 degrees and the patient's ability to reach the top of his head, and the time period is 2 weeks. In the second goal, the action or performance is increased strength, the measurable criteria are 4/5-strength grade and no demonstration of a significant trunk shift to the right, and the time period is 4 weeks. The reader should determine whether the third goal is properly written.

The PTA helping the patient to accomplish the first goal sees that the desired improvement in flexion needs to be met in 2 weeks. The PTA can plan each treatment session to include appropriate exercises and activities that will increase the flexion range of motion. The PTA will guide the exercises accordingly, monitoring progress by measuring the range of motion and observing the patient's attempts to touch the top of his head. At 2 weeks, the goal is that the patient is able to perform left shoulder flexion through the range from 0–110 degrees and reach the top of his head. The PTA can report to the PT and record achievement of the goal in the progress note.

The anticipated goals shown in Figure 7–1 also contain the qualities that demonstrate proper formulation and writing. In Situation A, the performance goals are moving up and down in bed, rolling from side to side, and reaching for the telephone and call bell. The measurable criterion is standby assist, and the time period is 2 weeks. In this case, the PTA can

---

A. Situation: Patient had stroke (CVA) 2 weeks ago and is now home, receiving physical therapy 3 times a week through a home health agency. His wife is the caregiver.

Dx: R CVA.

PT Dx: L hemiparesis with dependent mobility in all aspects.

Expected functional outcomes: At anticipated discharge date in 1 month.

1. Patient will ambulate with an assistive device and minimal assist for balance to the bathroom and to meals in 3 weeks.
2. Patient will be able to manage two steps with an assistive device and a railing as well as car transfers for next visit to the doctor in 4 weeks.

Anticipated goals:

1. Pt. will consistently move up and down in bed and roll from side to side with SBA in 2 weeks.
2. Pt. will consistently roll to L side and reach for telephone and call bell with SBA in 3 weeks.
3. Pt. will consistently move from supine to sitting on edge of bed and return to supine position with minimal assist to help swing L leg into bed in 1 week.
4. Pt. will consistently move from sitting to standing and back to sitting from bed, toilet, wheelchair, and standard chair with minimum assist for balance, control and even weight-bearing cuing in 2 weeks.
5. Using a quad cane, pt. will consistently ambulate bed to bathroom, and to meals with moderate assist for balance control and gait posture cuing in 1 week.

B. Situation: Patient is 1 week postoperation for total hip replacement and is in a subacute rehabilitation unit. Patient is receiving physical therapy 2X/day with plans to be discharged to home.

Dx: L total hip replacement

PT Dx: Weakened hip musculature and dependent in rising from sit to stand and ambulation.

Expected functional outcomes: At anticipated discharge in 20 days, patient will transfer and ambulate independently for return to home.

1. Patient will independently and consistently move from sit to stand and stand to sit using elevated toilet seat, and all other surfaces no lower than 18 inches.
2. Patient will independently and consistently walk with a straight cane on all surfaces and in the community.

Anticipated goals:

1. Pt. will consistently be able to sit to stand and return with SBA if boost is needed from edge of bed, elevated toilet seat, wheelchair, and standard dining room chair in 10 days.
2. Pt. will consistently be able to ambulate using a straight cane for balance on tiled and carpeted level surfaces, to bathroom and dining room for meals with SBA for balance control in 10 days.

Figure 7–1   Examples of expected functional outcomes and anticipated goals.

structure the treatment sessions to include instructions and practice in bed mobility, rolling, and reaching for the telephone and call bell. The PTA will help the patient progress by decreasing the amount of assistance provided until the patient can perform these movements with standby assist. In Situation B, the PTA will work with the patient to improve the patient's ability to move from supine to a sitting position on the edge of the bed (action). The PTA will help the patient progress by decreasing the level of assistance provided until only minimal assist is needed (measurable criterion). The PTA may choose to spend most of the treatment session time on this activity during the first week, because the time period for meeting this goal is just 1 week. These goals describe functional tasks and do not include other impairments, so a description of the patient performing the tasks with standby assist is the only measurable criterion needed. Goals could be written to include the quality of the movements or speed of the movement as other measurable criteria for these functional tasks.

Although the PTA does not design the functional outcomes or the anticipated goals, he or she can work with the PT by offering suggestions, notifying the PT when goals are met, and recognizing when the PT needs to modify or change goals. A PTA may write goals for each treatment *session* to help the PTA stay focused on the progression of the patient toward accomplishing the anticipated goals and the functional outcomes. The treatment *session* goals are the steps to accomplish the anticipated goals set by the physical therapist.

The PTA knows the patient's evaluation results and refers to the goals listed in the evaluation when writing the interpretation of the progress note data. This coordination of the evaluation and the progress note provides written proof of the PT-PTA team approach to the patient's care, thus enabling the reader to determine the quality of care being provided.

3-6-00   **Dx:** RUE lymphedema 2° mastectomy.
    PT Dx: Edema RUE limiting elbow ROM with inability to feed self and groom hair using RUE.
Pt. states she is able to move her arm and use it more to help dress herself and to adjust her bed covers.
Measurements taken before and after ICP/1 hr/50 lb/30 sec on 10 sec off/supine/RUE elevated 45° to reduce
edema.

	Before	After	3-4-00
Superior edge olecranon process	13"	12"	14"
3" above edge olecranon process	13.5"	12.5"	14.5"
3" below edge olecranon process	12.5"	11.5"	13.5"

All measurements read at superior edge of mark. Elbow flexion 0–95° today compared with 0–85° on
3-4-00. Observed pt. feeding self today using long-handled spoon in R hand. ICP effective in reducing
edema and allowing increased ROM in elbow flexion. Pt. making progress toward goal of decreased
edema and increased elbow room so pt. wil be independent in feeding and grooming hair without needing
assistive devices. Will continue ICP treatment per PT initial plan.
                                                                Richard Student, SPTA/JimTherapist, PT Lic #1063

Figure 7–2   Example of progress note describing a change in the impairment severity.

INTERPRETATION OF THE DATA CONTENT IN THE PROGRESS NOTE

Interpretation of the data is the most important section of the progress note. Most readers of the medical record look for this information first *because it tells the reader whether the physical therapy care is helping the patient.* It is the PTA's summary of the progress note data with comments about the relevance and meaning of the information. These comments inform the reader of the patient's response to the treatment *plan.* This is in contrast to the objective section, which records the patient's response to *each intervention.* The reader of the progress note is told whether the patient is making progress toward accomplishing the outcomes and goals. Any comment made by the PTA must be supported by the subjective and/or objective information. The comments should be grouped or organized so the information is easy to follow and understand.

Change in the Impairment

A summary of the meaning of measurements and test results or observations recorded in the objective data can describe a change in the impairment severity when this information is compared with the status of the patient at the initial evaluation. For example, if the objective data include girth measurements of the patient's arm that are less than previous measurements and the patient's elbow flexion measurements show greater ROM, the PTA can comment that the intervention has been effective in decreasing the swelling and thus improving the ability of the elbow to move (decreasing the severity of the impairment). See the example progress note in Figure 7–2.

Progress Toward Functional Outcomes and Goals

The PTA informs the reader about the patient's progress through comments about improvement in functional abilities and progress toward or accomplishment of the expected functional outcomes and anticipated goals. A statement about whether an outcome or goal has been met is documented in this section. The reader also can find a description of the patient's functioning in the objective data, which will provide evidence to support the PTA's conclusion about progress toward the outcome or goal (Fig. 7–3).

10-25-00   **Dx:** R CVA.
    PT Dx: L hemiparesis with dependent mobility in all aspects.
Pt. has been receiving PT twice a day for 3 days. Pt. able to lift buttocks with smooth motion 5X & scoot up
and down in bed, roll 5X independently to L side, roll to R side with minimum assist to bring L shoulder
over 5X. Pt. practiced 3X moving from sitting on edge of bed to sidelying on three pillows and returned to
sitting with minimum assist to initiate sidelying to sit 1X. Able to move from sit to stand and to return to sit
from edge of bed with bed raised to highest level, SBA for cuing for even wt. bearing, 3X. Pt. ambulated
from bed to bathroom to bed 3X using quad cane and moderate assist for balance and assist in advancing L
leg 2X. Pt. circumducts L leg due to inability to flex knee during pre-swing. Pt. making progress toward
goals of independent bed mobility, sit to stand with SBA and ambulation with quad cane and minimum
assist. Will consult with PT about adding exercises for knee flexion with hip extended to improve gait next
session. Jane Doe, PTA Lic. #2961

Figure 7–3   Evidence in the data information that supports the PTA's conclusion about progress toward the goal.

4-17-00   **Dx:** Bulging disc L4.
      PT Dx: Muscles spasms of R paraspinals limiting ability to tolerate sitting.
      S: Pt. states she still cannot sit more than 10 minutes. States she feels better if she keeps walking or moving. _____
      O: Massage/10 min/prone over one pillow/R paraspinal muscles L2–S1/to relax spasm followed by ice massage same area, to anaesthesia (7 min) to inhibit spasm with minimal change in muscle tone palpated. Pt. performed 10 press-up exercises and lay 5 min prone on elbows. Sat to watch body mechanics video but observed standing and pacing after 10 min. Sitting tolerance 10 min, same as last treatment session. _____
      A: No change in muscle tone with treatment, no change in sitting tolerance. Wondering if patient needs anti-inflammatory medication or a change in PT treatment plan. _____
      P: Will recommend PT re-evaluate and possible need to refer back to physician. _____
      Alice Alert, PTA Lic. #6240

Figure 7–4   An example of a progress note in which lack of progress is reported and recommendations are made.

Lack of Progress Toward Goals

Lack of progress or ineffectiveness of an intervention or the treatment plan is acknowledged and comments are made about the complicating factors. The PTA may offer suggestions and indicate the need to consult the PT. Again, there should be subjective or objective information to substantiate the PTA's conclusion or opinion. Figure 7–4 is an example of a progress note reporting lack of progress and offering recommendations.

Inconsistency in the Data

Sometimes there is an inconsistency between the subjective information and the objective information. The PTA calls the reader's attention to this in the interpretation of the data content. For example, a patient may report a pain rating of 9 on a scale of 1 to 10, 10 meaning excruciating pain. The PTA may observe the patient moving about in a relaxed manner, using smooth movements with no demonstration of pain behaviors or mannerisms. This inconsistency is noted, and the PTA may want to include possible suggestions as to what to do. Again, this is a good place for consultation with the PT (Fig. 7–5).

3-19-00   **PT Dx:** Anterior rotation of right ilium limiting sitting and stair climbing tolerance. Patient states she has been doing her home exercises regularly, can sit 45 minutes now, but still has pain when attempting to step up with her right leg. Reports feeling unsafe when carrying her 18-month-old daughter up the stairs. Rates her pain 7/10 before and after treatment. Pt. has been seen for three sessions. Direct contact US/1 MHz/vigorous heat/10 min/prone/right PSIS/to relax muscle spasms and prepare ligaments for mobilization. Pt. correctly performed muscle energy self-mobilization techniques to move ilium posteriorly. (See copy of instructions in chart.) Equal leg length observed supine and long sitting after US & mobilization, uneven leg length during same test before tx. Unable to palpate muscle spasms or level of PSIS due to patient's obesity. Patient correctly demonstrated her home exercises (see copy in chart), and used correct body mechanics to minimize right hip flexion when reviewing safe technique for picking up her baby. Ambulates with an antalgic limp, shorter step length and stance time on the right. Unable to step up on 7-inch stair with right leg, due to reporting too much pain. Sat with good posture, relaxed, minimal weight shifting 45 minutes watching nutrition video and waiting for her "ride." As patient was leaving the clinic, observed her climbing into her pick-up truck by stepping up with her right leg and using smooth, quick movements. This looked like it required approximately 80–90° hip flexion. Goal of 45-minute sitting tolerance met. Progress toward outcome of safe stair climbing without railing and using step-over-step pattern appears 0% in the clinic. Performance in the clinic of good sitting tolerance but poor stair climbing tolerance is inconsistent with patient's pain rating, equal leg length test, and observed performance outside the clinic. Will consult PT as to what should be done next treatment session. Pt. has two more treatment sessions scheduled. Puzzled Assistant, PTA Lic. #439

Figure 7–5 Documentation of inconsistent information in the data with reference to PT consultation.

1-17-00 PT Dx: Decreased walking tolerance due to R quad tendon repair.
S: Pt. states eager to walk with cane, no c/o. _____

O: tx: Respond E-stim./distal end R quad/supine/15 min/motor response/for muscle re-education. Pt. performed three sets of 15 reps of each of following strengthening exercises in supine: quad sets, terminal knee extensions, AROM hip abd./add., SLR. Pt. ambulated 150 ft from bed to down hall, tiled level surface, with single end cane in LUE, contact guard assist for sense of balance and security. _____

A: Decreased quad strength, decreased control with knee extension ex. Concern with problem of no superior excursion with max. attempt of quad set. At max. attempt, patella is able to be shifted med. & lat. Suspicion of scarring & adhesion on R quad tendon. _____

P: More balance work with SEC. Cont. tx 3X/week. Will consult PT about patella concerns. Pt. will see physician at 1st of next week. Mary Smith, PTA Lic. #346

Figure 7–6   Progress note with assessment statements that are not supported by information in subjective or objective data, or both.

The PTA should be cautious when documenting inconsistencies, because this information may be interpreted as accusing the patient of lying or faking the injury or illness. The subjective and objective data should indicate clearly that something "isn't right." The PTA should also confirm the inconsistency when interpreting the data. The inconsistency may indicate that the patient should be referred to another health-care provider or have the treatment plan revised.

Common Student Mistakes When Documenting the Interpretation of the Data Content

Comments such as "pt. tolerated treatment well" and "pt. was cooperative and motivated" are commonly found in documentation. These types of comments are to be avoided unless they are relevant to the content of the entire progress note and are supported by the subjective and objective data. This information is better presented through descriptions and measurements of the patient's response and functional abilities.

Students commonly comment about something that is not mentioned previously in the note. Sometimes a topic is documented that appears to "come out of nowhere." Again, evidence in the subjective or objective data must be present to support the interpretation of the data. Figure 7–6 is an example of a note with information that is not supported by data in the note.

It is not unusual to see students' notes that do not mention the goals or provide any comments about whether the patient is accomplishing the outcomes or goals. Comments tend to be only about the data that measure the impairment severity level and about the treatment procedures. Figure 7–7 illustrates this type of mistake.

3-5-00   Dx: Fx R humerus, cast removed 3-3-00.
PT Dx: Limited elbow ROM with inability to reach above second button from top, face, or hair.
S: Pt. states his arm seems to be getting stronger, as he can lift a 5-lb bucket of water. _____

O: Elbow ROM:

	before tx	after tx
flexion	40–115°	37–119°
pronation/supination	0–10° both	0–14°

All other UE ROMs WNL. _____

Skin that was under cast still dry and flaking, color WNL, no pressure areas evident. Wlp/102°F/20 min/RUE/to relax arm muscles, debride dry skin, and prepare for exercise. Pt. performed AROM exercises per instructions,10 reps each elbow flex/ext, forearm pronation/supination in water during last 10 min of treatment. Following wlp, pt. correctly demonstrated home exercise program to increase elbow ROM and strength (see copy in chart). _____

A: Moist heat and exercise effective in increasing elbow ROM.
P: Will consult PT about discontinuing whirlpool after tomorrow's session and will progress difficulty of exercises. Four more tx sessions scheduled.
                                    Jim Jones, SPTA/Mary Therapist, PT (Lic. #007)

Figure 7–7   A progress note that does not mention the goals, but confines comments only to the data that measure the impairment severity level and the treatment procedures.

SUMMARY   The interpretation of the data portion of the PTA progress note provides a summary of the subjective and objective information, thereby making the data meaningful. Comments are made about the patient's progress and the effectiveness of the treatment plan. This section must always contain statements describing the patient's progress toward accomplishing the outcomes and goals listed in the initial evaluation. It coordinates the initial evaluation with the progress notes to demonstrate PT-PTA communication, teamwork, and continuum of care. The PTA may make suggestions and report information that should be brought to the PT's attention.

All statements in this section must be supported by the subjective or objective information. The same rules previously discussed about subjective and objective content also apply. Topics in this section should be organized and easy to read. All information must be relevant to the treatment plan and the patient's problem.

REFERENCES   1. American Physical Therapy Association: Guidelines for Physical Therapy Documentation. APTA, Alexandria, VA, 1998.
2. American Physical Therapy Association: Guide to Physical Therapist Practice. APTA, Alexandria, VA, July 1999, Appendix 1-2.

➤ REVIEW EXERCISES

1. Explain why the interpretation of the data section of the PTA progress note is the most important section to most readers of the note.

2. Describe the difference between the expected functional outcome and an anticipated goal.

3. List three criteria for a properly written outcome or goal.

4. Explain the PTA's role in writing the outcome or goal.

5. List the content topics to be included when interpreting the data in the PTA's progress note.

6. Describe how each topic identified in item number 5 above is related to the initial evaluation to demonstrate the effectiveness of the PT's treatment plan.

7. List the most common mistakes that students make when writing the interpretation of the data portion of the progress note.

Practice Exercise 1 ➤

Goals should describe an action or performance, have measurable criteria, and have a time frame within which the goal is expected to be accomplished. Use the expected functional outcomes and anticipated goals in Figure 7-1, circle the action or performance, draw a line through the time period within which the goal is expected to be accomplished, and underline the word or words that suggest how to measure the performance or determine that the goal is met. The first goal is done as an example:

Patient will (ambulate) with an assistive device and <u>minimal assist for balance to the bath room and to meals</u> ~~in 3 weeks~~.

Practice Exercise 2 ➤

The following goals do not follow the criteria for writing goals correctly. They do not tell the reader much about the functional outcome of the patient.

A. *First, rewrite each goal so it contains an action (verb), can be measured, and establishes a time period for accomplishing the goal.*

B. *Second, use your imagination and rewrite each goal so it relates to a specific functional outcome or activity.*

1. Increase right knee PROM to 0–90°.

_____

_____

_____

_____

2. Sit on edge of bed in 3 days.

_____

_____

_____

_____

3. Ambulate 30 ft using standard walker in 4 days.

_____

_____

_____

_____

4. Increase strength of hip abductors from 3/5 to 4/5.

_____

_____

5. Decrease pain rating on pain scale from 6/10 to 3/10.

_____

_____

_____

_____

6. Return to work.

_____

_____

_____

7. Decrease pain with movement in 1-2 weeks.

_____

_____

_____

_____

8. Decreased edema in right thumb to allow active ROM to be WNL.

_____

_____

_____

_____

9. Able to step down a 4-inch step with no pain complaints.

_____

_____

_____

_____

10. Able to lift 10 lb from floor with 4/10 pain rating to allow occasional picking up infant son from floor in 4 weeks.

_____

_____

_____

_____

Practice Exercise 3 ➤ *The correctly written anticipated goal or expected functional outcome should have an action verb, measurable criteria for judging the quality of the performance of the action, and a time period for accomplishing the goal/outcome, and should relate to a functional outcome.*
    Critique the following goals and outcomes. Identify what is missing if a goal is not written correctly.

Increase gait training to 90 feet, 4 trials, rolling walker, standby assist in 2 weeks.

_____

_____

_____

Improve left shoulder flexion to 0–110°.

_____

_____

_____

Pivot transfer wheelchair to bed minimum assist.

_____

_____

_____

Gain right ankle dorsiflexion PROM to 0–15 in 4 weeks.

_____

_____

_____

Ascend and descend stairs with single-end cane.

_____

_____

Strength gain in left gluteus medius in 3 weeks.

_____

_____

_____

Transfer wheelchair to floor 3 out of 5 times in 6 weeks.

_____

_____

_____

Ambulate independently with forearm crutches bed to dining room for all meals in 3 weeks.

_____

_____

_____

Lift 35-lb boxes from floor to shelf in 4 weeks.

_____

_____

_____

Able to perform 3 sets of 10 reps leg presses with 150 lb, consistently controlling the movement so the knees do not hyperextend and the weight plates to not clang.

_____

_____

_____

(Answers to Practice Exercise 3 are in the Instructor's Guide)

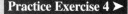

Practice Exercise 4 ➤   *Read the following progress note. Underline the subjective and objective data statements that support or provide evidence for the comments in the A section.*

> 4-17-00   **Dx:** R Colles' fracture, healed, cast removed.
>
> ――――――――――――――――――――――――――――――――――――
>
> **PT Dx:** Restricted ROM in wrist with inability to open doors, limited ability to grasp and pull for dressing activities.
>
> ――――――――――――――――――――――――――――――――――――
>
> **S:** Pt. reports able to put on pantyhose today without help from husband and turned bathroom doorknob to open the door.
>
> **O:** Pt. has been seen 2×. Pt. performed AROM exercises R forearm pronation/supination while in arm whirlpool, 110°F, 20 min, to increase circulation and increase extensibility to R wrist tissues to prepare for stretching exercises. Contract-relax stretching techniques, 5 reps each, to increase pronation, supination, and wrist extension ROM, sitting with forearm supported on table. Pt. correctly demonstrated home exercise program for strengthening finger flexion, wrist flexion and extension, and forearm pronation and supination (see copy in chart). ROM today vs. 4-10-00:

	4-17-00	4-10-00
R pronation	0-50°	0-40°
R supination	0-70°	0-60°
Wrist extension	0-30°	0-20°

> Grip strength 20 lb today, 10 lb 4-10-00. Pt. turned door handles and opened all inside doors in the clinic using R hand, but unable to turn handle and open door to outside. Able to grasp rope on scale and pull, exerting 3-lb force (2-lb 4-10-00).
>
> **A:** Strengthening and stretching treatment procedures effective in increasing strength and ROM, improving progress toward goals of independent dressing activities and ability to open all types of doors.
>
> **P:** To see pt. on 4-24-00 and notify PT discharge eval. to be 4-31-00. Will work on opening outside doors next visit.
>
> ―Sally Citizen, PTA, Lic. 5631

Practice Exercise 5 ➤   *Look at Figure 7–6. It illustrates documentation of information in the A section of this SOAP-organized note that is not mentioned in the subjective or objective sections. There is more in this note that does not constitute quality documentation. Critique the A section, and list what needs to be documented to make this a well-written progress note.*

(Answers to Practice Exercise 5 are in the Instructor's Guide)

Practice Exercise 6 ➤   *You are on your last clinical affiliation at XXX Rehabilitation Center, where they use the SOAP format for documentation. Your patient is Jim, who has quadriplegia as a result of a spinal cord injury from a snowmobile accident. When he tries to sit, he faints because blood pools in his paralyzed legs, causing his blood pressure to drop (orthostatic hypotension). You have been working on a tilt-table treatment plan to overcome the orthostatic hypotension and to accomplish the anticipated goal of ability to tolerate the upright position for 30 minutes. The functional outcome is for Jim to be able to sit for 2 hours. It is Friday afternoon, and you are writing your weekly progress notes. Interpret the subjective and objective data in the A section for this incomplete note. Write in black ink.*

108

1-20-00 **Dx:** Orthostatic hypotension 2° SCI C7.

_____

PT Dx: Unable to tolerate upright sitting.

_____

S: Pt. continues to c/o dizziness when he attempts sitting.

O: Pt. has had 3 sessions on the tilt table to develop tolerance for upright sitting.

First session BP dropped from 130/80 mmHg to 90/50 mmHg p 10 min at 40° elevation. Today BP dropped from 130/80 mmHg a tx to 100/60 mmHg p 15 min on tilt table at 50°. BP 125/75 mmHg 5 min p pt. returned to supine position.

A: _____

_____

_____

_____

Practice Exercise 7 ➤ *You are on your second clinical affiliation at XXX Hospital and have been working with Sally, who burned her L hip. You give her whirlpool treatments daily so the moving water will débride (i.e., clean out) the wound, and you use sterile technique to change the dressing. The goal is to promote healing of the wound so she will be able to sit properly and begin walking. You are writing your progress note after today's treatment session. Write the interpretation of the data portion of this incomplete note. Use black ink.*

11-2-00 **PT Dx:** Open wound due to 2nd-degree burn on L gluteus medius, not able to sit with even wt. bearing.

_____

Pt. reports itching around edge of wound. Pt. sat in whirlpool 100°, 20 min, for wound débridement and to increase circulation for healing, sterile technique dressing change. No eschar, edges pink, 1 tsp. drainage, clear, odorless. Diameter R outer edge to L outer edge: 4 cm today compared with 4-3/4 cm 10-31-00. Pt. sat in whirlpool with even weight bearing on pelvis and taking support from arms on edge of whirlpool.

_____

_____

_____

_____

_____

_____

_____

_____

Write the interpretation of the data portion of this note:

Dx: Subacromial bursitis R shoulder.

PT Dx: Pain c/o, ROM deficit in all shoulder motions, and strength deficit in anterior and middle deltoid limiting ability to load luggage into trunk of taxi and work as a taxi driver.

Expected Functional Outcome: Able to consistently load luggage into the trunk of the taxi with 0-3/10 pain rating in 10 days.

Anticipated Goals:

Pain rating reduced from 8/10 to 5/10 with shoulder movements for lifting and carrying objects in 5 days.

Consistent use of proper body mechanics using legs and minimizing shoulder motion for lifting, reaching, and carrying in 5 days.

AROM of all movements of the shoulder will increase by 50% of the AROM measured in the initial examination for lifting, reaching, and carrying in 5 days.

Subjective and objective information from your treatment session.

4-17-00

Pt. reported he was able to lift a passenger's brief case today with no pain, guessed the brief-case weighed about 15 lb; rated his pain with shoulder flexion 6/10 before ultrasound and 4/10 after the ultrasound treatment. Pt. has not missed any appointments. This is the 4th visit. Direct US/subacromial bursa/sitting with shoulder extended/forearm resting on pillow/1 w/cm^2 /8 min/to increase circulation and decrease inflammation. Pt. correctly followed home exercise instructions for AAROM "wand" exercises for R shoulder using a cane (see copy in chart). AROM (R) shoulder flexion 0-120° (0-80° initial exam). Initiated body mechanics training for reaching into trunk of car; needed frequent verbal cues to keep arms close to body and weight shift with legs. Consistently demonstrated proper form for squatting and lifting, no verbal cueing needed (occ cues needed last visit for keeping head and shoulders up). Able to lift 30 lb from floor 5× (20 lb 5× last visit).

a. What would you write next in the interpretation of the data section?

_____

_____

_____

b. Are the subjective and objective data recorded correctly?

_____

_____

_____

c. Are the goals written correctly?

_____

_____

Write the interpretation of the data section of this note:

Dx: 4 weeks status post surgery for herniated disc C4–C5.

PT Dx: ROM deficit all cervical motions limiting ability to look around and over shoulders for safe driving.

Expected Functional Outcome: Able to return to safely driving in 2 months

Anticipated Goals:
AROM cervical rotation (B) will improve 0–45° to be able to see objects at shoulder level in 2 weeks.
Independent in performing HEP of cervical AROM exercises to be able to look over shoulders in 1 week.

S: Pt. reports having difficulty with "chin tuck exercises" at home, notices she can see more items on the wall in the garage when she tries to look over her shoulder.

O: Pt. has been seen 3 times. Passive manual stretching, all cervical motions, 30 sec hold, 5 reps, supine, to increase ROM. Pt. gave correct demonstration of all exercises in HEP (see copy in chart) but needed correction and cueing to pull occiput toward ceiling with "chin tuck" exercises. Quality of the exercise improved after 10 reps. Cervical AROM (B) rotation 0–30° before stretching, 0–35° after stretching (0–20° initially).

A: _____

_____

_____

_____

_____

a. Are the subjective and objective data written properly?

_____

_____

_____

b. Are the goals written properly?

_____

_____

_____

Write the interpretation of the data portion of this note:

Dx: L lower extremity bone cancer with above-knee amputation.

PT Dx: L hip flexion/extension ROM deficit, L hip abductor strength deficit limiting ability to walk safely with prosthesis.

Expected Functional Outcome: Independent ambulation in home and community with prosthesis and appropriate ambulation aid in 1 month.

Anticipated Goals:
Hip flexion/extension PROM 0–110°, hip hyperextension 0–10°.
L hip abductor strength increase to lift 10 lb, 3 sets of 10 reps in 1 month.
Ambulation with cane on carpet, grass, steps in 2 weeks.

Pt. states he is able to lie prone with one thin pillow under abdomen instead of two pillows for 1 hour. Missed yesterday's session because of the flu. This is pt's 5th session. HP/L iliopsoas/20 min/to increase elasticity to prepare for stretching. Hip flexion PROM 15-110° before HP, 10-110° after HP. Contract-relax active stretching/L hip flexors/5×/prone/to gain hip extension ROM. PROM hip flexion 5–110° after stretching (20–110° initial exam). Required frequent reminders to breathe while performing 10 reps active extension exercises, prone over one pillow. Exercise performed with effort, movements not smooth. Required occ verbal cueing to maintain L leg in midline while performing L hip abduction strengthening exercises, side-lying, using 4-lb cuff weight (up from 3 lb last visit), 3 sets of 10 reps, exerting effort last 3 reps and tending to hold breath. Provided written instructions (see copy in chart) and 4-lb cuff weight for this exercise to be continued at home. Gait training on grass with quad cane on R (walker initial exam) requiring contact guard assist for safety with uncertain balance due to slight hip-flexed posture, uneven strides with shorter stance time on L.

a. Write the interpretation of the data information next.

_____

_____

_____

b. Are the subjective and objective data written correctly?

_____

_____

_____

c. Are the goals written correctly?

_____

_____

_____

(Answers to Practice Exercise 10 are in the Instructor's Guide)

Writing the Content: Intervention Plan

LEARNING OBJECTIVES

After studying this chapter, the student will be able to:
➤ Compare and contrast the plan content in the evaluation with the plan content in the PTA progress note
➤ Discuss how the plan section incorporates the PT–PTA team approach to patient care

INTRODUCTION

The previous chapters have shown how the examination/evaluation and progress note tell a story about the patient's physical therapy medical care. First, the patient's thoughts or contributions to the information are presented. Then, the objective facts are gathered and documented. Next, the information is summed up and given meaning. Finally, a plan is outlined telling the reader what interventions are proposed for the patient. This information is contained in the P section in the SOAP-organized note, the E section of the DEP model, and the second P section in the PSPG outline.

INTERVENTION PLAN CONTENT

The content in the plan section is more detailed in the physical therapy evaluation than the plan content in the progress notes. APTA's *Guidelines for Physical Therapy Documentation*[1] states that treatment plans "shall be related to goals and expected functional outcomes, should include the frequency and duration to achieve the stated goals."

Plan Content in the Evaluation

The PT outlines the intervention plans designed to accomplish the anticipated goals and expected functional outcomes. These plans are documented in the plan section of the initial evaluation. The treatment is directed toward the physical therapy diagnosis and includes two parts: (1) physical therapy activities or interventions that treat the impairments contributing to the patient's functional limitations, and (2) training in the functional tasks described in the goals and outcomes. The PT's plan will include treatment objectives. Written the same way as goals, objectives contain action words (verbs), are measurable, and have a time frame. They document the rationale for each activity or intervention listed in the plan. Figure 8–1 provides three examples of documentation of intervention plans.

INTERVENTION PLAN #1

Dx: R hip trochanteric bursitis.

PT Dx: Hip abductor muscle weakness and discomfort limiting tolerance for walking and stair climbing required at work.

Expected Functional Outcome: To be able to walk from car in parking lot to office and to climb two flights of stairs without using a railing in 4 weeks for return to work.

Anticipated Goals:
1. To be able to walk equivalent of two blocks with minimal hip abductor limp and 3/10 pain rating in 3 weeks.
2. To be able to climb one flight of stairs using railing and with 3/10 pain rating in 3 weeks.
3. To be able to increase hip abductor muscle strength to 5/5 in 4 weeks.

Intervention:
1. Ultrasound to R trochanteric bursa, moderate heating effect, to increase circulation to decrease inflammation and discomfort.
2. Exercises, including home program, for hip abductor muscles to strengthen to grade 5/5.
3. Home program of structured, progressive walking and stair climbing activities to increase tolerance to the activities without aggravating the bursitis.

US and exercise 3X/week for 2 weeks, then 2X/week for 2 weeks with emphasis on self-management and monitoring of home programs and discontinuation of US. Pt. has appointment with physician in one month. Rehab potential is good.

INTERVENTION PLAN #2

Dx: Fractures of L olecranon process and L hip.

PT Dx: Immobility required to allow healing causing patient to be dependent in ADLs, transfers, and ambulation so is unable to return to home.

Expected Functional Outcome: At discharge time, patient will be able to transfer and ambulate with support for return to home.

Short-term Functional Outcomes:
1. To be able to transfer from bed <--> chair <--> toilet with SBA in 2 weeks.
2. To ambulate with platform walker for support on L from bed to bathroom, and 200 ft to be able to ambulate required distances in the home with SBA in 2 weeks.
3. To be able to ascend one step using walker and SBA to enter home in 2 weeks.

Intervention Plan:
1. Exercises to strengthen all extremities to aid transfers and ambulation. Exercise plan to include home program.
2. Training and practice for transfers from all types of surfaces as required in the home.
3. Gait training with platform walker on level tiled and carpeted surfaces and one step as required in the home.
4. Home assessment visit to clarify needs for transfer and gait training planning.
5. Educate patient and family on hip protection and safety precautions for safe functioning in the home.

Pt. to be treated bid for 2 weeks with discharge to home with support and continued physical therapy through home health agency. Rehab potential good.

INTERVENTION PLAN #3

Dx: 4 weeks post fractures of L olecranon process and hip with healing in process.

PT Dx: Limited ROM and strength in L elbow and hip causing patient to be confined to ADLs within her home and requiring SBA.

Expected Functional Outcome: Discharge plan is for patient to be able to transfer and ambulate independently in her home environment, and to join family for summer activities in motor home on lake.

Short-term Functional Outcomes:
1. To ambulate independently using single-end cane within the home in 3 weeks.
2. To ascend and descend stairs using single-end cane and the railing independently in 2 weeks.
3. To walk to the end of the dock using single-end cane and SBA to sit and fish in 3 weeks.
4. To climb steps into motor home using single-end cane and SBA in 3 weeks.
5. To perform home exercise program independently and accurately in 1 week.

Intervention Plan:
1. Home program of exercises to increase ROM and strength of L elbow and hip in preparation for ambulation with cane and independent ADLs.
2. Transfer and ambulation training with progression of assistive devices appropriate for safe change from platform walker to goal of single-end cane.
3. Ambulation training on grass and dock using assistive device.
4. Stair climbing training with assistive device and railing in home and into motor home.
   Home health physical therapy 3X/week for 2 weeks and decrease to 2X/week for 1 week. Rehab potential is good.

Figure 8–1   Three examples of documentation of intervention plans.

As the patient's status changes and goals are met, only the PT may modify or change the intervention plans. These changes are documented in the interim evaluations. The PTA may not modify the intervention plans without consulting the PT. Discharge evaluations contain the plans for any follow-up or further treatment that may be required.

When goals, functional outcomes, and treatment objectives are written correctly, the PTA can follow them easily to plan each treatment session and measure treatment effectiveness and the patient's progress toward meeting the goals. (See Chapter 7 for more information.)

Plan Content in the Progress Note

The plan content in the PTA's progress note contains brief statements about the following:

1. What will be done in the next session to enable the patient to progress toward meeting the goals
2. When the next session is scheduled
3. What PT consultation or involvement is planned
4. Any equipment or information that needs to be ordered or prepared before the next session
5. The number of treatment sessions remaining before discharge

These statements typically contain verbs in the future tense. The verbs describe what will happen between now and the next treatment session or what will happen at the next session.

A comment about something specific the PTA wants to be sure to do at the next session goes in the plan section. This written comment serves as a self-reminder for the PTA (e.g., "Will update written home exercise instructions next visit," or "Will check skin over lateral malleolus this PM after patient has worn new AFO 6 hours"). It is also a way to inform another therapist who may be treating the patient next session.

When commenting elsewhere in the note about concerns, suggestions, or something that must be brought to the PT's attention, a statement is written in the plan section to indicate that the PT will be consulted or contacted (e.g., "Will consult PT about referring patient to social services"). This ensures follow-through, quality continuum of care, and PT–PTA communication. When the progress note is written by the PTA, the inclusion of such a statement in the plan section provides evidence of PT–PTA teamwork and collaboration. When the situation does not require consultation or immediate communication with the PT, the PTA can demonstrate PT–PTA teamwork by referring to the PT's goals or plan in the evaluation (e.g., "Will ambulate patient on grass and curbs this PM per PT's goal in initial eval.")

When the progress note is the method for keeping track of the number of treatment sessions the patient is receiving, the number of sessions to be scheduled is reported in the plan section. The objective data may state, "Pt. has been seen for physical therapy 3×." The plan portion of the note may read, "Pt. to receive 3 more treatment sessions," "Pt. has 2 more approved visits to be scheduled," or "Pt. will return on 2-16-00, 2-23-00, and anticipate discharge on 3-1-00."

Examples of PTA Plan Documentation

Additional examples of plan content statements likely to be read in a PTA's progress notes include the following:

- "Will increase weights in PRE strengthening exercises next session."
- "Will discuss with PT patient's noncompliance with exercise program."
- "Will consult with PT about adding ultrasound to treatment plan."
- "Will notify PT that patient is ready for discharge evaluation."
- "PT will see patient next session for reassessment."
- "Will ambulate patient on stairs this PM."
- "Will order standard walker to be available for treatment session on 8-4-00."
- "Will have blueprints for constructing a standing table ready for home visit on 9-11-00."

SUMMARY   The plan component of physical therapy documentation addresses what will happen during subsequent treatment sessions or in the future in general. The evaluations contain intervention plans and objectives designed by the PT to accomplish anticipated goals and expected functional outcomes. The PTA carries out the intervention plans designed by the PT, with notations to contact the PT when the plans need to be changed or modified. The PTA designs activities to help the patient progress within the guidelines described in the plans.

For the plan content in the progress notes, the PTA documents what is planned for the patient at the next session(s), telling the reader generally how the patient will make progress toward the goals. The plan section may also include (1) a reminder to do something more specific, (2) statements of intent to consult with the PT regarding any concerns or suggestions that were mentioned elsewhere in the progress note, and (3) the number of treatment sessions yet to be completed. A statement in the plan section that mentions communication with the PT reinforces and demonstrates the PT–PTA team approach to patient care.

REFERENCES   1. American Physical Therapy Association: Guidelines for Physical Therapy Documentation. APTA, Alexandria, VA, 1998.

➤ Review Exercises

1. Discuss what the reader will find in the plan section of the PT's evaluation.

2. Describe the PTA's role in designing the intervention plan.

3. Describe the content of the plan section of a progress note.

4. Explain how the plan section of the progress note can support the PT–PTA approach to patient care.

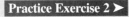

PRACTICE EXERCISES

Practice Exercise 1 ➤   *The progress note in Practice Exercise 6 in Chapter 7 is incomplete. Finish the note by writing the plan section, stating what you will do next. Use black ink and sign the note with your legal signature and your title (SPTA).*

_____

_____

_____

_____

_____

_____

_____

_____

Practice Exercise 2 ➤   *The progress note in Practice Exercise 7 in Chapter 7 is incomplete. Finish the note by writing the appropriate plan information. Use black ink and sign the note with your legal signature and your title (SPTA).*

_____

_____

_____

_____

_____

_____

_____

Practice Exercise 3 ➤   *Read the plans in Figure 8–1. Circle the activity or intervention and underline the measurable information. The first one is done as an example:*

(Ultrasound) to R trochanteric bursa, moderate heating effect, to increase circulation to <u>decrease inflammation and discomfort.</u>

What are the frequencies and durations (time periods)?

_____

118

Other Documentation Responsibilities

LEARNING OBJECTIVES

After studying this chapter, the student will be able to:
➤ Demonstrate adherence to the rule of confidentiality
➤ List two other documentation responsibilities shared by the PT and PTA
➤ Demonstrate proper documentation procedures when taking verbal physical therapy referrals over the telephone
➤ Demonstrate proper procedures, including documentation procedures, for releasing information about a patient's condition and treatment
➤ Explain what to do when the patient refuses treatment
➤ Demonstrate proper documentation procedures for completing and filing an incident report

INTRODUCTION

In addition to recording the physical therapy care of the patient, the PT and PTA share other documentation responsibilities. All clinical facilities have documentation procedures for recording telephone communications and for unusual events, such as patient refusal of treatment and incident reports. With all documentation, the rule of confidentiality must be followed.

THE RULE OF CONFIDENTIALITY

All medical records and information regarding the patient's condition and treatment are confidential. Only those providing direct care to the patient have access to this information. Any individual not providing direct care to the patient must be authorized by the patient to receive information about his or her medical care and condition. This is an ethical principle commonly called the *rule of confidentiality*.

The patient provides this authorization by signing a release-of-information form for each person or by naming each person. Figure 9–1 is an example of a release-of-information form.

The PTA may not provide information about the patient to anyone without first knowing whether the person is authorized to receive the information. Once authorization is obtained, then the facility's procedure for releasing information is followed.

Release of Information Form

Patient Name_____ DOB_____
Address:_____ Social Security # _____

I authorize and request XXX Medical Rehabilitation Center to release records maintained while I was a XXX patient, disclosing information as specified below. This form may be utilized for several parties to eliminate duplicate paperwork.

PURPOSE OF REQUEST:

__X__ Insurance Reimbursement   _____ Worker's Compensation
__X__ Subsequent Treatment/Intervention on behalf of patient   _____ Damage or claim eval. by attorney
_____ Other (Specify) _____

INFORMATION TO BE RELEASED:

__X__ Eval Reports   __X__ Discharge Reports
__X__ Progress Notes   __X__ Physician Order(s)
__X__ Plan of Care   __X__ Other (Specify)_____

By placing my initials in the appropriate space, I specifically authorize XXX to include in the records released, information relating to or mentioning the following, if any:

_____ Psychological conditions   _____ Drug or alcohol abuse

RELEASE:

*1. Release to: Physician   *2. Release to: Insurance Company
   Name: Name:
   Address: Address:

*3. Release to: Employer   *4. Release to: QRC or Disability Case Manager
   Name: Name:
   Address: Address:

5. Release to: Attorney Law Firm   6. Release to: Patient
   Name: Name:
   Address: Address:

7. Release to: 8. Release to:
   Name: Name:
   Address: Address:

*When a therapist requests courtesy copies, the above parties signified by an asterisk (*) will automatically receive copies of medical records.

REVOCATION

I understand that I may revoke this authorization at any time. If I do not expressly revoke this authorization sooner, it will automatically expire 1 year from the date of this authorization; or under the following conditions:

   a.) authorization may extend beyond one year if this is a worker's compensation case.

   b.) other (specify)

COPIES

A photocopy of this authorization X may   may not be accepted by you in place of the original.

SIGNATURE

Signature of patient or person   Date
authorized to sign for the patient

If signed by someone other than the patient, state how authorized

REFUSAL

I do not wish to authorize release of information to the following individual party(ies)

Name of party or parties

Signature   *Date*

Figure 9–1 Example of a Release-of-Information Form

The patient's medical record is kept in a secure location, such as behind the nursing station counter or in an office, to prevent unauthorized persons from reading it. The PTA respects this rule of confidentiality by returning the patient's medical record to its proper location or by passing it on to another authorized person only. The record must never be left lying unattended on a counter or desk. Any discussion about the patient's condition must occur in private areas and only with the patient, caregivers, and those authorized to receive the information.

Any researcher who wants to gather information from the medical record must also have the patient's permission. The researcher cannot publish or reveal the patient's name or any other descriptions that would identify the patient.

The Patient's Rights

Although the health-care facility is the legal owner of the medical record, the patient has the legal right to know what is in it. The patient must follow the facility's procedure to access his or her record. Usually the procedure simply involves asking the patient to sign a request form. PTAs need to be knowledgeable about the facility's procedure.

TELEPHONE COMMUNI-CATIONS

The PTA may participate in three common types of telephone conversations requiring documentation in accordance with the facility's policies and procedures: (1) taking verbal referrals for physical therapy treatment from another health-care provider; (2) receiving information about the patient from the patient or a representative of the patient; and (3) receiving inquiries about the patient's medical condition or about the physical therapy treatment from interested persons.

Referrals for Physical Therapy

Referrals for physical therapy services may be telephoned to the department by other health-care providers or their staff. Telephone orders for physical therapy services may be made by a physician, or by a nurse or receptionist acting under the physician's direction. One PT may call and refer a patient to another PT with expertise in the treatment of a particular patient's condition. Another health-care provider may telephone a referral because physical therapy is the more appropriate medical treatment for the condition of his or her patient. When receiving a referral over the telephone, the PTA should follow the facility's procedure for documenting the call.

Carrying a pen and notebook in your pocket at all times allows quick note taking when answering the telephone. Take notes to gather the information to document later. Each facility should have a procedure or form for recording telephone referrals. A copy or a similar form with the information from the call is sent to the referring provider for signature. This signature proves that the conversation and referral did take place.

Typically the documentation requirements for a telephone referral include the following:

1. Date of the call.
2. Name of the person phoning in the referral. You will know with whom to talk if any questions arise later.
3. Name of the health-care provider if the call is someone other than the provider, such as the physician's receptionist.
4. Name of the PTA answering the telephone and receiving the verbal referral. Again, it is important to know who can clarify questions.
5. Details of the referral and accompanying information regarding the patient.
6. Comment regarding plans to send written verification of the telephone referral to the referring provider.
7. Comment indicating that the referral will be brought to the attention of the PT.

Information From or About the Patient

The PTA may answer the telephone when a patient or family member calls to report a change in the patient's condition or ability to keep a therapy appointment. If the call is about a change in the patient's condition, the PTA may need to refer the caller to the PT or the patient's physician. If it is an emergency situation, the caller is advised to transport the patient to the emergency room or call 911. Documentation about this call may include:

1. Date and time of the call
2. Name of the person calling

3. Name of the PTA taking the call
4. A summary of the conversation, including the response of the PTA
5. A comment regarding the apparent emotional state of the caller (tone of voice, disposition, orientation)

Requests for Information About a Patient

Often persons other than those providing direct patient care have an interest in the patient's condition and treatment and may telephone to inquire about the patient's progress. Attorneys, insurance representatives, parents of children less than 18 years of age, and other relatives, friends, and neighbors are examples of persons who might call the physical therapy department. For example, a patient who was injured while working may have lawyers, a rehabilitation manager, an insurance representative, and an employer, all of whom may want to know about the patient's medical care. When the PTA answers the telephone and the caller asks about a patient's condition, the PTA must follow the rule of confidentiality.

PATIENT REFUSAL OF TREATMENT

As discussed in Chapter 2, after receiving information about all aspects of the treatment the patient or a representative of the patient must consent to the treatment plan; this consent may be informal and verbal or formal and written. This policy and procedure ensures that the patient is not being coerced into any course of action. When the patient gives a verbal consent, the PT documents the consent in the initial evaluation. An informed consent document should contain the following[1]:

1. A description of the physical therapy diagnosis and the proposed intervention plan written in language that the patient or representative of the patient can understand
2. Name and qualifications of the responsible PT and other physical therapy personnel likely to be providing the care
3. Any risks of or precautions to the treatment procedures that the patient should consider before deciding to agree to or refuse the treatment
4. An explanation of any alternative treatments that would be appropriate, including risks or precautions that need to be considered if the alternative treatment is used
5. The expected benefits of the proposed treatment plan and the expected outcomes if the physical therapy problem is not treated
6. Responsibilities of the patient or representative of the patient in the intervention plan
7. Answers to patient's questions

The patient does have the right to disagree with the plan or to change his or her mind later and refuse treatment. When a patient refuses treatment, there are several things the PTA can do:

1. Use active listening skills, interview, and talk with the patient to try to determine the reason for refusal. The patient may have a very good reason why it would not be appropriate to receive treatment at that time. I vividly remember a gentleman in a nursing home who refused therapy 1 day without explaining why. After spending some time talking with him, he revealed that his dog had passed away the previous evening. This man was grieving his loss and would not have been able to concentrate on his therapy activities.
2. If there does not seem to be a reason for the refusal, make sure the patient fully understands the purpose of the treatment and the expected outcomes if the problem is not treated.
3. If the patient continues to refuse, recognize the patient's right to refuse, document this in the patient's chart, and notify the PT.

Documenting Treatment Refusal

The PTA documents, in the medical record instead of the progress note, the patient's statement of refusal and reason. The PTA describes his or her response and action taken. A statement about notifying the PT is included. The documentation may read as follows:

8-3-00

1:00 PM: Pt. refused treatment this PM. After being encouraged to attend at a later time, pt. stated her sister was visiting from out of state, and the only time she would be able to visit with her was this afternoon. She expected her soon and anticipated the visit would last all afternoon. Agreed to cancel treatment this PM and scheduled pt. for tomorrow AM. Will inform PT.

—Bob Smith, PTA

THE INCIDENT REPORT

An *incident* is anything happening to a patient, employee, or visitor that is (1) out of the ordinary, (2) inconsistent with the facility's usual routine or treatment procedure, or (3) an accident or situation that could cause an accident. All medical facilities should have a policy and procedure for documenting incidents in an *incident report*. During the first or second day of internship or on a new job, the student or the newly employed PTA should read the clinic's instructions for completing and filing an incident report.

Purposes of the Incident Report

The incident report is used for risk management and legal protection. Following the policy and procedure for reporting incidents protects everyone who uses the facility (i.e., all patients, employees, and visitors) from future incidents. The procedure describes a method for providing a prompt response to medical needs, identifying and eliminating problems, and gathering and preserving information that may be crucial in litigation. The report contains information that identifies dangerous situations that either caused or could cause an injury.

Risk management uses this information to change the situation, thereby reducing the risk for injury. The incident report alerts administration and the facility's lawyer and insurance company to the possibility of liability claims. It "memorializes important facts about an alleged incident that create a record for use in further investigation" (p 183).[1]

Legal Responsibility When an Incident Occurs

Only the eyewitness fills out and signs the incident report. If more than one person witnessed the incident, one of the eyewitnesses completes the report but includes the names of the other witnesses. The person documenting the incident must follow the facility's procedure.

The incident report is completed on a form unique to the facility. Most medical facilities use similar forms, which typically ask for the following information:

1. *Name and address of the person involved in the incident:* When the person involved is an employee or visitor, his or her home address is given. If the person is a patient, the address, date of birth, gender, admission date, and patient status before the incident are provided. The patient's medical diagnosis and physical therapy diagnosis are recorded along with a brief summary of the care the patient has received.
2. *An objective, factual description of the incident:* The PTA completing an incident report does not express an opinion, blame anyone or anything, or make suggestions as to how the incident might have been prevented. The incident is to be described as the eyewitness saw it, not as someone else described it. No secondhand information is to be included in the report. The circumstances surrounding the incident, the condition of the affected person after the incident, and the course of action taken are described.
3. *Identification of all witnesses to the event:* The report includes addresses of the witnesses, if known, as well as identification of equipment involved by model number and manufacturer.

Each facility has a time period within which the report should be submitted. This can vary from 24 hours to 3 days after the incident. Because the incident report is not considered part of the medical record, it is placed in a file separate from the patient's medical record. The PTA must document the incident in the patient's chart. However, the PTA does not mention that an incident report was completed. The report is a confidential, administrative document for use in case of litigation and risk-management review and action. Box 9–1 summarizes the "do's and don'ts" of incident reporting.[2] Figure 9–2 is an illustration of a completed incident report. The names and the situation are fictitious.

1. **DO** notify your PT.
2. **DO** know your facility policy and procedure for reporting an incident.
3. **DO** write legibly and use professional terminology.
4. **DO** include names and addresses of employees or visitors who know anything about the incident.
5. **DO** give the completed report to your supervising PT to route for the necessary signatures.
6. **DON'T** mention that you've filed an incident report in the patient's chart.
7. **DON'T** photocopy an incident report.
8. **DON'T** write anything in the report that implicates or blames anyone for the incident.
9. **DON'T** use incident reports for disciplinary actions.
10. **DON'T** use the report for complaining about co-workers or other employees.
11. **DON'T** talk about the incident with noninvolved personnel. Remember *CONFIDENTIALITY.*
12. **DON'T** acknowledge any incident or give any information until you've checked with your PT or a supervisor.

Adapted from Documentation. In Clinical Pocket Manual. Nursing 88 Books. Springhouse Corporation, Springhouse, PA, 1988, pp. 135-136.

PREDISPOSING CONDITIONS

Diagnosis: Fx Ⓡ hip   hypertension

Mental Status (i.e., Oriented, Alert/Confused, etc.): -alert & oriented

List pertinent medications if applicable: Tylenol   lanoxin   tenex

Follow up measures to Incident:

MD & family notified, vital signs checked every 2 hours for 12 hours

Was a Medical Device Involved?   ☐ Yes   ☒ No   Manufacturer's Name and Address (if Available on Equipment or Packaging):

Type _____ Model No. _____

Serial No. _____ Lot No. _____

Incident Reported By: Joan Anderson   Title: PTA

| Date of Report: 11/21/00 | Signature & Title of Person Preparing Report: Joan Anderson/PTA |

Reviewed by DON: Virginia McDormel/Rn (Signature)   Reviewed by Administrator: Mike Bond (Signature)

Date: 11/22/00   Charted: ☒ Yes ☐ No   Date: 11/23/00

Reviewed by Medical Director: Dr Steve Jones (Signature or initials)   Date: 11/30/00

DO NOT WRITE BELOW THIS LINE-TO BE COMPLETED BY ADMINISTRATOR/DON

Vulnerable Adult Report Made?   ☐ Yes ☒ No

Incident Reported To (Circle as many of the following as applicable.):

Local Welfare Agency   Local Police Department   County Sheriff's Office   Office of Health Facility Complaints

Other (Explain) _____

Date Report Called in (Within 5 Days): _____ Approximate Time: _____ ☐a.m. ☐p.m.

Name of Person Spoken to: _____ Reported By: _____

Date Report Mailed: _____ To Whom: _____

incident.rep

Figure 9–2 An example of the front and back of a completed incident report. The names and situation are fictitious.

```
┌─────────────────────────────────────────────────────────────────────────────┐
│                          ABC HEALTH CENTER                                    │
│                           INCIDENT REPORT                                     │
├───────────────────────────────────────┬───────────────────────────────────── │
│ Resident/Visitor #1   Jane Doe         │ Resident/Visitor #2    n/a           │
├───────────────────────────────────────┼───────────────────────────────────── │
│ Address:  7700 Grand Ave.              │ Address:                             │
│           Duluth                       │                                      │
│                                        │                                      │
│ Phone #: 628-2341    DOB 1/17/17       │ Phone #:           DOB               │
├───────────────────────────────────────┼───────────────────────────────────── │
│ Date: 11/21/00    Time  2:30   am/pm   │ Location of Incident: P.T. Dept      │
└───────────────────────────────────────┴───────────────────────────────────── ┘
```

Description of Incident:

                    Pt was standing in parallel bars with PTA holding on with transfer belt,
Pt performing ®L/E standing exercise, she became pale and dizzy, could not walk back to chair,
was lowered to floor by PTA. Never lost consciousness, felt much better once reclined. With
assist of RPT was lifted into w/c

Assessment: Describe injury (if any) in detail:

      Skin tear on ® forearm when arm hit bar while lowering small 1.5X 2.0 open area
      with small amount of blood

Name/Title of All Witnesses:	Safety Measures in Use:
Mary Smith/RPT	Transfer Belt: __X__
Joan Anderson/PTA	Siderails: _____
	does not
	Restraint: use____ Type:_____

Intervention: None Required _____   At Facility _X_____

Describe:

      Vital signs checked and charted in nursing chart, skin tear was cleansed & protective
      covering in place. ROM to U/E & ⓛL/E WFL s̄ pain! ®L/E ROM within hip precaution
      limits s̄ pain

Resident #1

Hospitalized: Yes ____ No _X_	Date _n/a_ Time ____ am/pm	Hospital _n/a_
Physician Name: Harvey Jones	Notified by: Dana Olson/RN Date 11/21/00 Time 3:00 am/pm
Family Name: Robert Doe/son	Notified by: Dana Olson/RN Date 11/21/00 Time 3:15 am/pm

Resident #2 n/a

Hospitalized: Yes ____ No ____	Date ____ Time ____ am/pm	Hospital ____
Physician Name:	Notified by:	Date ____ Time ____ am/pm
Family Name:	Notified by:	Date ____ Time ____ am/pm

Figure 9–2   *Continued.*

SUMMARY   The PT and PTA are responsible for documenting numerous events and tasks occurring during the course of a day. The PTA must know the facility's procedures for documenting various types of telephone conversations, documenting patient refusal of treatment, and completing incident reports. General descriptions of these common events and their procedures were discussed in this chapter.

REFERENCES   1. Scott, RW: Legal Aspects of Documenting Patient Care. Aspen, Gaithersburg, MD, 1994, pp 123–125, 183.
2. Clinical Pocket Manual: Documentation, Nursing 88 Books. Springhouse Corp., Springhouse, PA, 1988, p 135.

➤ Review Exercises

1. List three documentation responsibilities other than writing progress notes that are shared by the PT and PTA.

2. Describe the rule of confidentiality.

3. Discuss methods the PTA uses to adhere to the rule of confidentiality.

4. Discuss the purpose of a release-of-information form.

5. Describe the information that the PTA should document when taking a telephone referral for physical therapy services.

6. Explain why the name of the caller and the name of the PTA taking the call should be documented when a referral is telephoned to the physical therapy department.

7. Discuss how the PTA should respond when the patient refuses treatment.

8. Explain how the PTA should document refusal of treatment.

9. Define an *incident*.

10. List the information typically included in an incident report.

11. Explain how an incident report benefits the patient, employee, and visitor.

12. Explain how an incident is documented in the patient's medical record.

Practice Exercise 1 ➤ *Read the following scenario in which the patient refuses treatment. Document this in the form of a progress note.*

You are a PTA working in a long-term care facility. You treat Janet Smith, in Room 102, daily for lower-extremity strengthening exercises, transfer training, and gait training with a walker. Ms. Smith has peripheral vascular disease with decreased circulation to her legs. She has become generally weakened because of bed rest while a small open wound on her right heel healed. You see her twice a day, and this is the third day of treatment, 11-15-00. As soon as you enter her room, she tells you she cannot have therapy today because her "right leg is too sore and swollen from being up in the wheelchair too long." You see that she is in bed, both legs elevated, T.E.D.s* (antiembolism stockings) on, and you do not observe any significant increase in edema around the lateral malleolus. She has consistently had minimal edema around the lateral malleolus. After discussing the importance of moving her legs and using her muscles to increase her circulation, you cannot convince her to participate in the therapy session. You remind her to continue doing her isometric exercises for her legs as she had been instructed when she was on bed rest, and you leave to check the nursing notes in her medical record. You see that the nurse has charted that the patient did request an increase in her usual dosage of Tylenol, which is ordered as needed. You will notify the PT and plan to see Ms. Smith tomorrow.

_____

_____

_____

_____

_____

_____

_____

_____

_____

_____

_____

PROGRESS NOTE OT____ PT____ SLP____	
Name:_____ Room #_____ MR# _2001_ Date_____	

This therapist has observed at least every 6th treatment   Signature_____
delivered by the assistant and deems it to be appropriate.
        ___MS___

_____

*Kendall Health Care Products, 15 Hampshire St, Mansfield, MA 02048

Read the following scenario, which describes a situation that requires an incident report. Because you are the eyewitness, you must fill out the report. After completing the report, identify the safety lesson to be learned as a result of this incident.

You are a PTA working in a long-term care facility. You are in your patient's room working on transfer training from his wheelchair to the bed, which has wheels. Your patient is Mr. X, 75 years old, who had fractured his right hip and underwent hip repair with a prosthesis. He is allowed 40 lb of partial weight bearing and is learning to use a walker. He is alert and oriented and otherwise is in good health. The only medication he takes is Tylenol, as needed. The plan is for him to be discharged to his home, where he lives with his 70-year-old wife. It is Friday, December 1, 2000, 10:20 AM. Mr. X stands from the wheelchair and proceeds to do a standing pivot transfer with the walker to get into bed. You have the transfer belt on him and you are standing on his right side. As he turns, his left knee buckles and he starts to fall. You guide him down onto the bed, but the bed rolls back and you must lower the patient to the

INCIDENT REPORT	
Resident/Visitor #1:	Resident/Visitor #2:
Address:	Address:
Phone #: DOB_____	Phone #: DOB_____
Date: Time_____ am/pm	Location of Incident:
Description of Incident:	
Assessment: Describe injury (if any) in detail:	

Name/Title of All Witnesses:	Safety Measures in Use:
	  Transfer Belt:_____
	  Siderails:_____
	  Restraint:_____ Type:_____

Intervention: None Required _____ At Facility _____	
Describe:	

Resident #1			
Hospitalized: Yes___ No___	Date_____ Time_____am/pm	Hospital_____	
Physician Name:	Notified by:	Date_____Time____am/pm	
Family Name:	Notified by:	Date_____Time____am/pm	
Resident #2			
Hospitalized: Yes___ No___	Date_____ Time_____am/pm	Hospital_____	
Physician Name:	Notified by:	Date_____Time____am/pm	
Family Name:	Notified by:	Date_____Time____am/pm	

PREDISPOSING CONDITIONS

Diagnosis:

Mental Status (i.e., Oriented, Alert/Confused, etc.):

List pertinent medications if applicable:

Follow-Up Measures to Incident:

Was a Medical Device Involved?   ☐ Yes   ☐ No   Manufacturer's Name and Address (If Available on Equipment or Packaging):

Type_____   Model No._____

Serial No._____   Lot No._____

Incident Reported By:_____   Title:_____

Date of Report: Signature & Title of Person Preparing Report:

Reviewed by DON:_____   Reviewed by Administrator:_____
         (Signature)   (Signature)
         Date:_____
Date:_____   Charted: ☐ Yes ☐ No

Reviewed by Medical Director:_____   Date:_____
         (Signature or Initials)

DO NOT WRITE BELOW THIS LINE - TO BE COMPLETED BY ADMINISTRATOR/DON

Vulnerable Adult Report Made?   Yes ☐   No ☐

Incident Reported To (Circle as many of the following as applicable.):

Local Welfare Agency   Local Police Department   County Sheriff's Office   Office of Health Facility Complaints

Other (Explain)_____

Date Report Called In (Within 5 Days):_____   Approximate Time:_____ ☐ a.m. ☐ p.m.

Name of Person Spoken to:_____   Reported By:_____

Date Report Mailed:_____   To Whom:_____

floor. You rest his head and trunk in your lap, call for help, and notice that his legs are positioned straight in front of him. He denies having pain in his right hip or leg, but does complain of pain in his right buttock. He is nervous and anxious. The nurse, Jane Doe, and a nursing assistant, Tom Jones, hear you and come running. With their help, you are able to lift Mr. X up and into bed. The resident in orthopedic surgery, Dr. Young, happens to be in the building. He is called and is able to examine Mr. X immediately. He doesn't think there has been any damage to his hip and believes the buttock pain may be due to bumping against the side rail as he was lowered to the floor. Nursing will monitor the skin condition and his pain complaints, and Mr. X will rest in bed for the remainder of the day.

Safety Lesson: _____

_____

Documentation Summary: Study Guide

The previous nine chapters in this book have objectives, review exercises, and practice exercises to help the reader learn the information. This chapter presents important points from the book in an outline format for quick reference and for use as a study guide.

I. **Introduction to Documentation**
   A. Definition of documentation.
      1. A legal record of the patient's medical care from admission to discharge.
      2. Written proof authenticating care given to the patient.
      3. A written record holding the caregiver accountable for the quality and cost of care.
      4. The rationale supporting the medical necessity for treatment.
   B. The evolution of PT and PTA responsibilities.
      1. Changes in physician referral methods have influenced PT and PTA treatment and documentation responsibilities.
         a. Referrals used to read like a prescription, telling the therapist exactly what to do. A therapist was considered a technician providing physical therapy treatments.
         b. As PTs began to educate physicians about the capabilities of PTs, referrals changed to read "evaluate and treat."
            (1) PTs needed evaluation skills to examine and identify the patient's problems that could be treated with physical therapy.
            (2) PTs documented the physical therapy evaluations.
            (3) First PTA school opened in 1967. The PTA was viewed as the technical health-care provider administering physical therapy treatments under the direction and supervision of the PT.
         c. Direct access allowed the consumer to seek physical therapy services without a referral from the physician; available in Nebraska since 1957, in California since 1968, and in Maryland since 1979. Today only five states do not have direct access language in their state practice acts.
            (1) Additional responsibility of the PT to recognize a patient's signs and symptoms not treatable by physical therapy and refer the patient to more-appropriate health-care providers.
            (2) Increased PTA responsibility to team up with the PT in observing and documenting the patient's response to treatment.
      2. The establishment of Medicare (Health Insurance for the Aged and Disabled Act) in 1965.

---

* Review questions are not applicable for this chapter. The reader will find practice exercises after the study guide.

a. Additional documentation standards were established, making caregivers accountable for justifying treatment.

b. Stage set for documentation standards and criteria established by federal and state governments and various agencies.

3. Limited dollars available for health care.

a. The major factor influencing the treatment and documentation responsibilities of the PT and PTA.

b. Necessitates the identification and use of the most effective and efficient PT treatments.

c. Contributes to the scrutiny of medical records by insurance companies to identify and support the practice of providing quality medical care as efficiently as possible and at a reasonable cost.

d. Makes proper documentation a must to reflect effective and efficient care.

4. Effectiveness of physical therapy care measured by how well the patient can function in his or her environment; documented in the description of the patient's functional abilities.

C. The role of documentation in ensuring quality of care.

1. Facilitates good communication among caregivers; the method by which all the patient's health-care providers communicate with one another..

2. Provides the basis for reimbursement decisions; third-party payers will not reimburse for treatment procedures that are not deemed appropriate or effective.

3. Supplies information or data for research activities (e.g., physical therapy research designed to determine efficacy of physical therapy treatment procedures).

4. Following documentation standards and criteria defined by the following:

a. Federal government (Medicare).

b. State government (Medicaid, medical assistance, workers' compensation, state physical therapy practice acts).

c. Professional agencies (e.g., APTA).

d. Accrediting agencies (e.g., Joint Commission on the Accreditation of Health-care Organizations, Commission on Accreditation of Rehabilitation Facilities).

e. Individual health-care facilities.

5. Follow the documentation standards by *following the facility's procedures.*

II. Documentation Content

A. Information in the medical record is grouped into six general content categories.

1. Data: All information that relates to why the patient is seeking medical help and the patient's response to the medical care provided.

a. Subjective data: Information gathered through an interview of the patient or a representative of the patient; information that is told to the caregiver.

b. Objective data: Information gathered by the health-care provider through an examination; information that can be measured, reproduced, or observed by another health-care provider with the same training.

2. The problem requiring medical treatment: Data are analyzed to identify the problem that requires medical treatment.

a. Medical diagnosis: Identification of a systemic disease or disorder determined by the physician's examination.

b. PT examination of the patient, evaluation of data, and determination of the physical therapy problem/diagnosis.

c. Physical therapy diagnosis: Anatomical abnormalities and dysfunctions (impairments) interfering with the patient's ability to function in his or her environment.

d. Incorporation of the patient's impairment with his or her functional limitations.

3. Treatment plan or action: Plan of action to treat the problems.
   a. Action outlined in the medical record.
   b. Information given to patient about the treatment plan.
   c. Informed consent by patient or representative necessary before the plan is initiated.
4. Goals and functional outcomes, or purpose of the treatment plans documented.
   a. Purpose of the treatment plan.
      (1) Gives direction to the medical care.
      (2) Provides a means of measuring the effectiveness treatment.
   b. Outcomes with functional focus.
   c. Patient-oriented outcomes.
5. Record of administration of the interventions in the treatment plan via daily or weekly progress notes.
6. Treatment plan effectiveness.
   a. Information about the patient's response to the interventions, and the interpretation of that information.
   b. Most important information in the medical record to answer the question, "Is the treatment plan appropriate and effective?"

B. Documentation responsibilities.
   1. PT responsible for documenting the examination and evaluation reports.
   2. PTA primarily responsible for writing the progress notes; task shared with the PT.

C. Physical therapy examinations and evaluations.
   1. The PTA may assist the PT in performing an examination.
      a. Take notes for the PT.
      b. Help gather subjective data.
      c. Perform tests in which he or she has been trained, such as goniometry, manual muscle testing, taking vital signs, and measuring girth.
   2. The PTA *may not* evaluate, interpret the examination data, identify the physical therapy problem, design or modify the PT intervention/treatment plan, or set treatment goals and outcomes.
   3. The PTA carries out the PT's intervention plan and assists the patient in accomplishing the treatment goals and outcomes.
   4. The PTA's role in the three types of physical therapy examination and evaluation reports:
      a. Initial examination and evaluation: Performed the first time the PT sees the patient. The PTA may not treat a patient who has not undergone a PT's initial examination and evaluation.
      b. Interim evaluations/documentation of continuum of care: These are performed periodically during the course of the physical therapy treatment sessions to measure the patient's progress and change or modify the intervention plan as indicated. The PTA writes progress or interim notes, but the PT documents interim evaluations.
      c. Discharge evaluation/summation of care: This is the final note about the patient, summarizing the interventions provided, evaluating the degree of plan effectiveness, and recommending further care if needed. The PT documents the summation of care reexamination and reevaluation.
   5. The PTA may write a discharge summary.
      a. The information is only a summary of the interventions provided and a description of the patient's status at discharge.
      b. The summary should not include an interpretation of the information or recommendations for further care after discharge.
      c. The PTA discharge summary cannot be the final note about the patient's care in the chart.

III. Organization of the Content

   A. The information in the medical record is typically organized according to the disciplines providing the medical care, the patient's problems, or a combination.

      1. The SOMR is organized according to the medical services the patient is receiving.

      2. The POMR is organized according to the list of problems being treated by the health-care providers.

   B. The content of the medical record can be organized in a variety of formats, each with its own logical arrangement of components.

      1. At present, SOAP organization is the most common format for arranging the information.

         a. S stands for subjective; this section contains the subjective data.

         b. O stands for objective; this section contains the objective data.

         c. A stands for assessment; this section contains the interpretation of the data and identification of the problems, goal, and outcomes.

         d. P stands for plan, this section contains the treatment plan.

      2. The PSPG format is often used in progress notes that accompany a SOAP-organized examination and evaluation report.

         a. The P section contains the statement of the patient's problems.

         b. The S section contains the status of the patient at the time of the note, including the subjective and objective data.

         c. The P section contains the plan for future treatment sessions.

         d. The G section contains the goals/outcomes, with statements about progress, any goals/outcomes accomplished, and any new goals/outcomes set.

      3. DEP is another recommended documentation format.

         a. D stands for data, and contains subjective and objective data.

         b. E stands for evaluation, and contains the interpretation of the data, the problems, and the treatment plan.

         c. P stands for performance goals, and identifies the functional outcomes that the treatment is designed to accomplish. The goals/outcomes include a time frame for achievement.

      4. All the models for organizing the documentation content have a common thread. The PTA can adapt to any model when writing progress notes by following these guidelines:

         a. Introduce the progress note with a list or statement that tells the reader the physical therapy diagnosis about which the note is written.

         b. Next, provide the subjective data and objective data, comparing or relating it to the data in the PT's examination report.

         c. Discuss the meaning of the data as it relates to intervention plan effectiveness and the patient's progress toward accomplishing the goals and outcomes listed in the PT's evaluation report.

         d. Discuss the plan for future treatment sessions and involvement of the PT.

   C. The content can be presented in a variety of formats.

      1. Computerized documentation.

      2. Flow charts and checklists, used mainly by hospitals, rehabilitation centers, and nursing homes.

      3. Letter format, typically to the physician, commonly used by private-practice outpatient clinics.

      4. The IEP, used in schools.

      5. The cardex format, used within physical therapy departments to record current interventions. Interventions can be duplicated by another PT or PTA by following the information written on the cardex.

      6. Standardized Medicare forms for documenting patient status and seeking recertification for further treatment.

IV. Writing the Content: Guidelines

A. The focus of this text is on writing the progress note.

1. The progress note is the record of the interventions or treatment procedures administered and their effectiveness.

2. Typically, the progress note is written daily when the patient's condition is acute and weekly if the condition is more chronic. If the patient is seen intermittently (e.g., once a week, twice a week, three times a week), a note is written after each therapy visit.

3. The content of a progress note must include the following:

   a. Specific treatment provided, its purpose, and the patient's response to each intervention.

   b. Equipment provided or sold to the patient and any written instructions given to the patient.

   c. Patient status, progress toward goals and outcomes, or lack of progress, written in functional terms.

4. The organization of the content of the progress note must be in a form the facility uses.

5. The medical diagnosis and/or the physical therapy diagnosis may introduce the progress note.

B. Principles and guidelines for documenting in a legal record must be followed by everyone writing in a medical record, with documentation written as if writing a letter to a jury or to a lawyer, and following the legal guidelines.

1. Be accurate. Never falsify the information.

2. Be brief, using short and concise sentences containing relevant information.

   a. Use abbreviations minimally or not at all.

   b. Keep in mind that abbreviations can be misunderstood, resulting in dangerous situations.

3. Be clear.

   a. When describing the patient's function, use words to "paint a picture of the patient" so the reader can "see" the patient in his or her mind.

   b. Write legibly; sloppy handwriting suggests carelessness.

   c. Use correct punctuation, grammar, and spelling to demonstrate accuracy and care.

4. Date and sign all entries.

   a. Use your full legal signature.

   b. Place the initials of your title after the signature.

   c. Write your license number after your title initials to identify that the physical therapy intervention was provided by a qualified, trained physical therapy provider.

5. Use black ink (this guideline may change).

6. Do not allow opportunity for the record to be changed or falsified.

   a. Do not use erasable pens.

   b. Do not erase errors. Cross them out with one line, write the date and your initials above the error.

   c. Do not leave lines blank. Draw a line through any blank lines or large spaces.

   d. Be timely. Carry a notebook and pen in your pocket to take quick notes for accurate documentation later.

V. Writing the Content: Subjective Data

A. Description of subjective data.

1. Subjective data consist of information about the patient and the patient's condition that is told to the health-care provider by either the patient or a representative of the patient.

2. Subjective data in the progress note must be relevant to the patient's physical therapy diagnosis and treatment plan.

        a. While working with the patient, the PTA uses active listening, which includes analytic, directed, attentive, and exploratory listening.

        b. Relevant information is grouped in the categories of medical history, environment, emotions or attitudes, goals, functional outcomes, unusual events, chief complaints, response to treatment, and level of functioning.

     3. The complaints that cause the patient to seek medical help are the symptoms of the patient's condition, the subjective data.

  B. Organization and writing of the subjective content.

     1. The subjective data can be organized or grouped according to the content categories listed in V.A.2.b. when recording detailed data.

     2. The progress note does not have to contain subjective data. Subjective data is included only if the information is relevant to the effectiveness of the treatment interventions.

     3. Guidelines for writing subjective data:

        a. Use verbs such as states, reports, denies, says, and describes.

        b. Quote the patient directly to document clearly the patient's confusion, denial, attitude toward therapy, and use of abusive language.

        c. When information is provided by someone other than the patient, document who provided the information.

  C. Pain information in the subjective data section.

     1. Pain is perceived and described by the patient.

     2. It is best described in some form of a pain profile.

        a. Pain scale, usually numerical.

        b. Checklist of descriptive words.

        c. Body drawing and color codes.

     3. Pain profiles are always located in the subjective data section of the progress note.

VI. Writing the Content: Objective Data

  A. Description of objective data.

     1. Objective data consist of information about the patient's condition gathered by examination, testing, and observation.

     2. The information can be measured, reproduced, or observed by another health-care provider with the same training.

     3. The objective data include the signs of the patient's condition.

     4. Visual or tactile observations made by the PTA are objective data when another PT or PTA would see or feel the same information.

  B. Organization and writing of the objective data.

     1. The content organization flows from one topic to the next.

     2. Three categories of content:

        a. Results of measurements and tests.

        b. Description of patient's functioning.

        c. Description of interventions provided.

     3. Writing of the objective content guidelines:

        a. Repeat tests and measurements that were taken during the initial examination to record the patient's response to the treatment plan.

        b. Document the results so the reader can easily compare them with the results in the initial or previous examination reports or notes.

        c. Use words to describe the patient performing a function so the reader can picture the patient's functioning.

        d. Use words that portray the skilled services of the physical therapy provider.

        e. Write a description of the intervention provided in enough detail that another PT or PTA could read the description and duplicate the intervention. This detailed description can be found in the progress note and/or the cardex in the physical therapy department.

        f. Include the purpose of and patient's response to each intervention. This information will be useful for researching the most effective treatment procedures.

       g. Include a copy of any written information given to the patient.

       h. Mention any equipment provided or sold to the patient.

  C. Common student mistakes.

    1. Writing what they did and not what the patient did.

    2. Rambling or failing to organize the information by topic.

VII. Writing the Content: Diagnoses, Goals, Functional Outcomes, and Treatment Effectiveness

  A. Description.

    1. Interprets the data.

    2. Is most commonly considered assessment or evaluation information and included in the A section of the SOAP-organized report.

    3. Provides answers to the "what does it mean?" question a reader might ask after reading the data.

    4. Gives meaning to the data.

    5. Provides the rationale for the necessity of the skilled physical therapy services.

  B. Interpretation of the data in the PT evaluation.

    1. Identifies the physical therapy diagnosis based on the data.

    2. Lists expected functional outcomes relating to the treatment of the functional limitations.

    3. Lists the anticipated goals relating to the treatment of the impairments. Goals and outcomes:

       a. Describe the action.

       b. Have measurable criteria that determine their accomplishment.

       c. Include the expected time period for achievement.

  C. Interpretation of the data in the progress note.

    1. Comments about the effectiveness of the interventions and the treatment plan as a whole.

    2. Comments about the patient's progress toward accomplishment of the anticipated goals and ultimately the expected functional outcomes.

    3. Comments about lack of progress and any suggestions or recommendations to be discussed with the PT.

    4. All comments supported by evidence in the subjective and objective data.

    5. Evaluation of possible inconsistency between the subjective and objective data.

    6. Interpretation of the data is always related to the information in the PT's initial evaluation report.

  D. Common student mistakes.

    1. Vague comments about the patient's condition or progress.

    2. Comments not supported by evidence in the subjective or objective data.

    3. Tendency to forget to talk about the progress toward the goals and functional outcomes.

VIII. Writing the Content: Intervention Plan

  A. The plan content in the PT's initial evaluation report:

    1. Contains the intervention/treatment plan and objectives set by the PT.

    2. Serves several purposes:

       a. Provides a design to accomplish the goals and outcomes.

       b. Is directed toward eliminating or minimizing the impairments and functional limitations.

       c. Includes training in the functional tasks required to accomplish the functional outcomes.

       d. Cannot be modified or changed by the PTA.

  B. The plan content in the progress note:

    1. Tells the reader what the PTA will do at the next treatment session or between sessions.

    2. Indicates when the next session will be and how many more sessions are scheduled.

3. Includes a comment that demonstrates the PT's involvement, reinforcing the PT–PTA team approach to physical therapy patient care.
4. Uses verbs in the future tense.

IX. Other Documentation Responsibilities

A. Rule of confidentiality.
1. Only the persons directly providing patient care are permitted to have access to the patient's medical record. This is the rule of confidentiality.
2. The patient can authorize other persons to have access to his or her medical information by signing a release-of-information form for each person.
3. The PTA may not release any information about the patient to any unauthorized person.
4. The PTA is to discuss the condition of the patient only in private and only with authorized persons.

B. Patients' rights and documentation.
1. The patient has the right to know what is written in his or her medical record.
   a. The medical record is owned by the medical facility.
   b. The patient typically signs a form to access his or her medical record.
2. The patient has the right to consent to treatment.
   a. The patient is informed of all the details of the treatment plan.
   b. The patient consents either verbally or formally (in writing) to the treatment plan before it is initiated.
   c. Formal consent is made by the patient's signing an informed consent form with the PT (not the PTA) witnessing the signature.
   d. The verbal or formal consent is documented in the PT's initial evaluation report.
3. The patient has the right to refuse treatment.
   a. The patient may refuse a treatment session or refuse to continue treatment.
   b. Attempts are made to determine the reason for refusal by using active listening skills and talking with the patient.
   c. The patient must understand the purposes of treatment and the consequences of not being treated.
   d. A patient who refuses treatment is referred to PT.
   e. The PTA may need to allow the patient to refuse.
   f. The conversation is documented in the patient's chart.

C. Documentation of telephone conversations.
1. Verbal referral for physical therapy.
   a. Note data about the patient.
   b. Note name of the caller and name of the PTA taking the call.
   c. Note date and time of the call.
   d. Note that the referral will be brought to the PT's attention.
   e. Send a written copy of the information to the caller for signature.
2. When the patient or representative of the patient calls to report a change in the patient's condition:
   a. Refer the caller to the PT.
   b. Refer the caller to the patient's physician.
   c. Advise the caller to take the patient to the ER or to call 911.
   d. Document in the patient's chart the date and time of the call, the name of the caller, and the PTA taking the call, and describe the conversation, including the action taken by the PTA.
3. When someone calls asking about the condition of the patient:
   a. The PTA must follow the rule of confidentiality.
   b. When the PTA is unsure whether he or she should answer the caller's question, the PTA should refer the caller to the PT.

D. The incident report.
  1. An incident is anything out of the ordinary that happens to a patient, employee, or visitor. It is:
     a. Not part of the facility's usual routine, treatment procedures, or functioning of the equipment.
     b. An accident or something that could cause an accident.
  2. The incident is documented on the facility's incident report form.
     a. The form must be documented within the time period specified in the facility's procedure.
     b. Only the eyewitness writes the report.
     c. The report contains only written facts as they happened, including time, location, name of person involved, names and addresses of eyewitnesses, condition of the environment, equipment involved, condition of the person involved before and after the incident, and action taken.
     d. Opinions, accusations, and suggestions are not included.
     e. The eyewitness to the incident completes and signs the report.
  3. The incident report accomplishes several goals:
     a. Informs risk management of hazards and potential hazards that can be corrected.
     b. Alerts administration, lawyers, and insurance company representatives of the possibility of a liability claim.
     c. Protects the patient, employee, and visitor.
  4. The incident report is confidential.
     a. The report is placed in a special file, not in the chart.
     b. The incident is documented in the patient's chart, but no reference to the incident report is made in the chart.
     c. The report is a confidential, administrative document for use in case of litigation and risk-management review and action.

SUMMARY   The PTA is responsible for complete, accurate, and proper physical therapy documentation in the patient's medical record. All documentation should be clear to anyone who reads the chart, regardless of the reader's training. The PTA provides documentation primarily in the progress note, providing evidence that the PT's treatment plan is being carried out and that the plan is effective in improving the patient's level of functioning in his or her environment.

The theories and skills described in this text are illustrated in the PT's initial examination and evaluation report in Figure 10–1. The PTA's progress note relating to the initial examination and evaluation report is shown in Figure 10–2.

GUIDELINES FOR CRITIQUING THE PROGRESS NOTE

As you read and critique a progress note, look first at the organization to see if the writer:

1. Introduced the progress note with a list or statement that tells the reader the physical therapy diagnosis about which the note is written.
2. Placed the subjective and objective data first.
3. Compared or related these data to the data in the PT's initial examination report.
4. Discussed the meaning of the data in terms of intervention plan effectiveness and progress toward accomplishing the anticipated goals and functional outcomes listed in the PT's evaluation report.
5. Discussed the plan for future treatment sessions and involvement of the PT.

Next, look more closely at each content area.

1. Are legal guidelines followed?
   Black ink or typed?
   Legible?
   Error crossed out with one line?
   Error dated and initialed?

Name: Mrs. S.   **Physician:** Dr. R.
Facility: XXXX Nursing Home   **Date:** 4-22-00

Dx: Left humerus and left hip fracture.

Subjective: Pt. states she had fallen on bricks while at the St. Patrick's Day parade on 3-17-00. She saw Dr. R. on 4-21-00 when he removed the immobilizer and ordered the start of physical therapy. States she lives in senior housing where there are no steps for her to climb, has been independent, drove her car, and did all her household chores, cooking, and self care; wants to return to independent living. Past medical Hx: fractured R hip 12 years ago and was back to normal, everyday living without the use of an assistive device. Mastectomy on left 30 years ago and has swelling and pain in LUE since. Arthritis in both hips. Ccs: bladder infection, dizziness when first up in sitting, and nervousness and apprehension about therapy. Nursing reports pt. has not been up out of bed much for the past month due to her refusing.

Objective: Palpation revealed no tenderness to the lower extremity or the upper extremity. Pt. did have minimal swelling in the left ankle and mod. to max. swelling in the LUE at wrist and elbow (measurements not taken).

ROM (measured in supine)

	Active	Passive
L shoulder flexion	0° c/o pain	$0–95^\circ$
L should abduction	$0–55^\circ$	$0–90^\circ$
L shoulder ER	0°	$0–12^\circ$
L shoulder IR	WNL	WNL
L elbow flexion	WNL	WNL

Wrist and finger flexion slightly decreased by swelling. L knee flexion in supine $0–65^\circ$. MMT— L hip flexors 5-/5, L quads 4+/5, L hamstrings 5-/5, L shoulder flexors 2/5, L shoulder abductors 2/5, L shoulder IR & ER 4/5. Transfers —Able to perform standing pivot transfer wheelchair to mat with mod. assist for balance; pt. uses only RUE. Holds LUE in somewhat guarded position and unable to bear much wt. on LLE. Sit to supine with min. assist for control in lowering trunk; able to lift LLE. Supine to sit with mod. assist for raising herself (unable to use LUE to help), sit to stand with standby assist for balance. Independent stand to sit with LLE extended due to decreased knee flexion, but pt. sits on edge of bed, leans backward, and complains of dizziness. Ambulation—Pt. ambulated in hall on tiled surface with rolling walker, SBA for balance, 25 ft, wt. bearing as tolerated on left. L shoulder was depressed, as pt. was not bearing wt. on LUE.

Physical Therapy Dx: Decreased ROM, strength, and mobility secondary to a left humerus and left hip fracture requiring dependent transfers and ambulation.

Expected Functional Outcome: To return to independent living and to return to her previous lifestyle.

Anticipated Goals:
1. To increase strength to at least 4/5 in all LUE muscles to aid in transfers and ambulation in 2 months.
2. To increase ROM to WFL for all shoulder, hip, and knee motions to aid in transfers and ambulation in 1 month.
3. To perform independent transfers from bed, toilet, various heights chairs and ambulation with assistive device on tiled, carpeted, and sidewalk level surfaces in 2 months.
4. To perform home exercise program independently and accurately in 2 weeks.

Treatment Plan:
1. AROM and gentle stretching exercises to all shoulder, hip, and knee motions to increase ROM for transfer and ambulation activities.
2. Strengthening exercises for all UE muscles, including home program to aid transfers and ambulation.
3. Gait training with assistive device on tiled and carpeted level surfaces and on sidewalk.
4. Transfer training from bed <--> chair <--> toilet and from various heights and types of chairs and couches for independent functioning in the home.
5. Home assessment visit to clarify needs for transfer and ambulation training planning.

Pt. to be treated bid for 3 weeks and decrease to 1X/day, 5X/week for 5 weeks. Anticipate discharge to independent living at home in 2 months. Rehab potential good.

Mary Therapist, PT (Lic. #)

Figure 10–1   A physical therapy initial examination/evaluation.

5-18-00	**Dx:** L humerus & L hip Fx.
	PT Dx: Dependent transfers, ambulation, and limited knee ROM.
	S: Pt. states she sat in the lounge chair in her room last night without needing to extend her L leg because she could bend her knee more now; nurses upset with her because she walked Ⓘ in room with standard walker last night. Denies having dizziness.
	O: Contract-relax stretching/3 sets/4 reps/to gain L knee flexion/sitting in lounge chair. After tx, AROM L knee flexion 0–75°, PROM 0–80°, measured goniometry sitting (0–65° in initial eval.). Observed pt. Ⓘ sit to stand from lounge chair using R hand in center of walker, L hand on arm of chair. Ambulated min. assist for pt. sense of security, wide-base quad cane to protect LLE, lounge chair to nursing station (@ 50 ft), tiled surface, rest, and ambulated back. Needed assist for mild loss of balance recovery 1X. Observed pt. ambulate Ⓘ, standard walker, chair to bathroom, stand to sit, sit to stand from toilet, ambulate room to dining room (@ 100 ft), partial wt. bearing L.
	A: Improved knee flexion allows easier transfers from low chair and toilet. Progress toward STGs #2 and #3 in initial evaluation is 75%. Ready to be allowed independent ambulation with walker in room and on nursing floor.
	P: Will notify PT of Ⓘ amb. status with walker so nursing can be notified. Will continue to progress pt. with quad cane and add ambulating on carpeting tomorrow AM
	Jim Doe, PTA

Figure 10–2   A progress note relating to the initial examination/evaluation in Figure 10–1.

Note dated?

Complete legal signatures with titles?

Lines drawn through long blank spaces?

2. Are subjective data documented correctly?

Are they information told to the therapist?

Are they information relevant to the treatment session?

If pain is documented, is it in the subjective data section?

3. Are objective data documented correctly?

Is there a record of the number of treatment sessions completed and an explanation for any treatment sessions missed?

Is the information about the interventions sufficient to allow another therapist to duplicate the interventions?

Is the purpose of each intervention documented?

Is the target tissue or treatment area identified?

Is there a description about how the patient performs functional activities?

Can the reader clearly visualize the patient's performance; does the note paint a picture of the patient?

Does the note describe what the PT or PTA observed?

Was a copy of any written instructions or information given to the patient put in the chart?

Are measurements consistent with the measurements in the initial examination report?

Are measurements related or compared to previous measurements?

Is it evident that the interventions provided could be done only by a trained physical therapy provider?

4. Was data interpretation correct?

Does this section answer the "what does it mean?" question? Does it give meaning to the data?

Does the interpretation summarize the subjective and objective data?

Are there statements about the patient's progress toward accomplishing the anticipated goals listed in the initial evaluation report?

Are there statements about the patient's progress toward accomplishing the expected functional outcomes listed in the initial evaluation report?

Are any concerns or suggestions mentioned?

Are there statements that are not supported by the subjective or objective information?

5. Is the plan appropriate?

Does the information relate to what will happen next?

Is there information about the number of treatment sessions scheduled, the number remaining, and anticipated discharge?

Is there reference to the PT's plan, the PT's initial evaluation report, working with the PT, or consulting the PT?

Overall, does the note describe quality physical therapy care in such a manner that anyone reading the note will understand the information?

Copy the statements in the following narrative PTA progress notes under the appropriate categories.

PROGRESS NOTE 1

3-10-00

Pt. is disoriented. She states, "It is Christmas and I don't have my shopping done." Observed pt. scratching at her wound dressings. Pt. has a decubitus over L lat. malleolus interfering with ability to wear proper shoe for ambulation. Wound dressing half off upon arrival at dept. Wound measures 3 cm horizontally from outer edge to outer edge (4 cm initial eval.), loose necrotic tissue, no drainage. Foot whirlpool 104.8°F, loose tissue dislodged, and dressings changed. Will consult PT re: designing wrap over bandage to keep pt. from pulling dressing loose. 50% progress toward goal of clean, healing wound to prepare for ambulation.

—Sue Smith, PTA

PT Dx: _____

_____

Subjective Data:
S: _____

Objective Data:
O: _____

Interpretation of the Data:
A: _____

Plan:
P: _____

PROGRESS NOTE 2

2-10-00

Pt. ambulated 33 the length of the // bars (about 30 ft) $\bar{c}$ min. assist for sense of security, with verbal cues for posture and heel–toe stepping. He needs max. assistance for sit $\longleftrightarrow$ stand for strength to get up and for control when sitting down. Gluteus maximus and quads 3/5. Major mm groups in LEs 3/5 to 4/5 strength range. Pt. is not independent in ADL due to muscle weaknesses. Pt. states he wants to go home. Maximum assist for transfer bed $\longleftrightarrow$ commode $\longleftrightarrow$ w/c. Will continue to work to ↑ mm strength and try sliding board transfers this PM. Pt. demonstrated 3 reps each of LE strengthening exercises to be performed in the ward with wife's help (see copy in chart). Pt.'s wife says she cannot care for pt. at home. Pt. is 82 years old $\bar{c}$ terminal cancer.

PT Dx: _____

Subjective Data:

S: _____

_____

_____

Objective Data:

O: _____

_____

_____

Interpretation of the Data:

A: _____

_____

_____

Plan:

P: _____

_____

_____

Practice Exercise 2 ➤ *Place "Pr" next to statements that are physical therapy problems/diagnoses, "SD" next to subjective data statements, "OD" next to objective data statements, "ID" next to statements that interpret the data, and "P" next to plan statements.*

_____ Pt. reports pain relief several hours after treatment.

_____ Performed Codman's exercises with 2-lb wt. to distract shoulder.

_____ Electrode placed 2 inches above R elbow crease line.

_____ R hemiplegia with spasticity and dependence for transfers and ambulation.

_____ Will instruct in proper stair climbing next session.

_____ Missed 2 of his last 5 treatment sessions because of illness one day and refusal the other.

_____ C/o pain in RLE.

_____ Recommended family install railing on wall along stairs for safety.

_____ Goal met for child to roll side-lying to supine and prone 1/3 trials at least 33 in 2 months to improve mobility.

_____ Had terrible headache last night.

_____ Will await further orders from physician.

_____ Pt. able to demonstrate home exercise program with good form.

_____ Pain intensity increased from 5 to 6/7.

_____ Requires moderate assist to get up from w/c and to lift legs back into bed.

_____ States he needs to lift a maximum of 70 lb from floor to conveyor belt.

_____ Performed 10 reps of UED1 exercises on the R using red Thera-Band* and 20 reps of same exercise on the L with blue Thera-Band.

_____ Ambulated with forceful knee hyperextension during stance phase.

_____ My goal is to play golf.

_____ Atrophy of quads and gastrocs limiting ability to climb stairs.

_____ Will take standard walker to patient's home next visit.

_____ Wrist flexors 3/5, extensors 2/5 strength.

_____ Mother stated child rolled supine to prone last night.

_____ Decreased muscle tone palpable following massage.

_____ Progress toward goal of independent car transfers and community ambulation 80%.

_____ Pt. squats with narrow base of support and rounded low back, placing object in front of knees.

Practice Exercise 3 ➤ *Rewrite the following progress note so the information is in the correct (i.e., logical) sequence. Then use the Guidelines for Critiquing the Progress Note (see p. 139) and list the ways this note could be better written.*

3-26-00

Pt. has met his outcome of independent crutch walking. Says he needs to be able to climb three flights of stairs to get to his apartment. Will work on stair climbing next session. Handrail on L going up. Pt. crutch walked NWB, 300 ft on grass outside c̄ no assistance. R foot edema. Circumference equal L foot measurements. R knee flexion 10–110°. Pt. showing good progress in LE mobility.

—Jim Jones, PTA

_____

_____

_____

*Thera-Band Resistive Exerciser, The Hygenic Corporation, Akron, Ohio.

_____

_____

_____

This note could be better written if _____

_____

_____

_____

_____

_____

_____

Practice Exercise 4 ➤ *Critique each of the following progress notes. They all relate to the same medical diagnosis and physical therapy diagnosis.*

Dx: 1 month post R ankle sprain
_____

PT Dx: Limited R ankle ROM & strength interfering with ability to walk uphill to get to his house.
_____

Progress Note 1: 4-20-00

 S: Pt. states he's feeling better.

 O: Gave US. Instructed in home ex. program. Instructed in amb. with cane.

 A: Pt. tolerated tx well. Making progress.

 P: Continue tx

—S. Student, SPTA/Wary T. Sign, PT

_____

_____

_____

_____

_____

Progress Note 2: 4-20-00

 S: Pt. reports less pain when walking but continues to have difficulty walking uphill.

O: Gave US to ankle, 1.5 w/cm², 5 min to prepare for stretching. Did contract–relax stretching exercises, dorsiflexion 0–5°, plantar flexion 0–40° (i.e., dorsiflex 25°, plantarflex 5–35°). Pt. correctly performed home ex. program using red Thera-Band to strengthen dorsiflexors, toe rises for plantarflexors, and prolonged (30-min) stretch. See copy in chart. Pt. ambulated 100 ft, SEC, supervision for verbal cueing to minimize limp.

A: US & ex. effective in increasing ankle ROM. Pt. making progress toward goal of amb.

P: Continue per PT plan.

—Better Student, SPTA/Will Sign, PTA

_____

_____

_____

_____

_____

Progress Note 3: 4-20-00

S: Pt. states it is easier to walk. Reports increased pain when walking uphill.

O: Immersion US/R deltoid ligament, peroneus longus/brevis tendons/vigorous heat (1.5 w/cm²)/5 min/for stretching. Pain before tx 5/10, after tx 3/10. Contract–relax stretching for ankle ROM.

	4-15-00	4-20-00
Dorsiflexion	25°	0–5°
Plantarflexion	5–35°	0–40°

Pt. correctly demonstrated home ex. program to strengthen all ankle muscles for stability using 3 sets of 10 reps with red therapeutic band & prolonged (30-min) stretch positions to increase ROM. See copy in chart. Pt. ambulated with SEC, mild-steppage gait, with slight foot slap at initial contact. Quality of gait improved with verbal cues to decrease knee flexion and use the ankle ROM. Ambulated on level sidewalk and level, uneven grass.

A: Pt.'s progress toward goal of ① amb. in community with amb. aid = 80%. US & ex. effective in increasing ankle ROM and quality of gait.

P: Continue per PT initial plan.

—Good Student, SPTA/Will Sign, PT

_____

_____

_____

Progress Note 4: 4-20-00

Pt. describes a "stiffness" pain today following tx rated 3/10 vs. 5/10 before tx. States has difficulty walking uphill. PROM, 1 rep to assess all R ankle motions gives firm end feel. Slight softening of end feel after immersion US/1 MHz/vigorous heat (1.5 w/cm^2)/5 min/R deltoid ligament & peroneus longus & brevis tendons/pt. sitting/to increase elasticity, warm tissue to prepare for stretching. Contact–relax stretching, 3 reps each dorsiflexion & plantarflexion.

	4-15-00	4-20-00
Dorsiflexion	25°	0–5°
Plantarflexion	5–35°	0–40°

Pt. correctly demonstrated dorsiflexion & plantarflexion strengthening exercises using red Thera-Band, 3 sets of 10 reps, & 30-min prolonged stretch positions to increase ankle mobility per instructions in written home program. See copy in chart. Able to use blue Thera-Band 10 reps. Pt. ambulated one city block on level sidewalk & level, uneven grass surface, using single-end cane, with supervision for verbal cueing to decrease knee flexion and use ankle dorsiflexion during initial swing. Quality of gait pattern improved by last 100 ft of the walk. Continues to demonstrate shortened stance phase, mild antalgic gait. Pt. has been seen 4×. 90% progress toward goal of ① community ambulation with or without ambulation aid. Ankle ROM increasing and strength gains with progression to more resistance (blue Thera-Band). To be seen 4-25-00 & 4-30-00 (anticipated d/c session). Will add walking uphill next session. Will notify PT of possible d/c evaluation on 4-30-00.

—Best Student, SPTA/Super Therapist, PTA, Lic. #123

Practice Exercise 5 ➤ *Use the Guidelines for Critiquing the Progress Note (see p. 139 and critique the progress note in Figure 10–2.*

_____

_____

_____

_____

_____

_____

_____

Practice Exercise 6 ➤ *Rewrite and improve the progress notes in Chapter 4, Practice Exercise 3 (and continued in Exercise 5).*

_____

_____

_____

_____

_____

_____

_____

_____

Practice Exercise 7 ➤ *The following is a physical therapy initial examination/evaluation, followed by related exercises.*

HOME HEALTH PHYSICAL THERAPY EXAMINATION/EVALUATION

Patient's name: _____Mr. X_____ Physician: _____

Diagnosis: Failed R hip prosthesis, R total hip revision.

History: 71 YO man who underwent R total hip revision and hospitalization 7-5-00 to 7-11-00. Pt. stated on first night home that he dropped R leg too far over side of bed and experienced a "pop." Currently experiences more side effects from this episode, denies increased pain on weight bearing but reports pain with spasms in R hip/thigh. Is up at night with frequent urination. States he previously could walk independently without an ambulation device, did his yard work, and could drive. Has follow-up visit with Dr. in 2 weeks. He is retired and lives with his wife who states she is willing and able to assist him.

Physical Status: Communication—Pt. wears hearing aids, is difficult to understand because of decreased articulation, is oriented, has good attention span, has no memory deficits, is cooperative but presents with a flat affect. Palpation—Staples still in place in R hip incision, no derangement in hip noted. ROM—WFL in all joints except R hip flexion limited to 90° per total hip protocol and R hip abduction limited 25%. Moderate heel cord tightness noted. MMT—R hip abduction 22/5, flexion 32/5, requires assist for R SLR, R knee flexion/

149

extension 32/5, otherwise all WFL. Sitting balance good, standing balance fair and requires support of crutches, no problems with coordination.

Functional Status: <u>ADLs</u>—Ⓘ for feeding and hygiene/grooming, uses crutches, high chairs, and elevated toilet seat, needs assist for RLE when getting in/out of bed, taking a sponge bath, dressing lower extremities. Pt. ambulates with crutches and supervision limited distances within his home using a weight-bearing-as-tolerated pattern for R but does not bear wt. on heel. <u>Physical environment</u>—House with several steps to enter, low-pile carpet or tile throughout, single bed with bathroom down the hall.

Physical Therapy Diagnosis:

1. Decreased strength/ROM RLE interfering with transfer ability from bed and chairs. Dependent sit ↔ supine and bed mobility.
2. Limited crutch ambulation within home secondary to decreased RLE strength and endurance.

Expected Functional Outcomes:

1. Safe and Ⓘ transfers from variety of surfaces in home in 3 weeks.
2. Safe and Ⓘ household ambulation with appropriate ambulation device for 5 or more min, up/down stairs to exit home in 3 weeks.
3. Wife/pt. to carry out home exercise program correctly and Ⓘ in 1 week.

Intervention Plan:

1. Home program of ROM and strengthening exercises to increase ROM and strength of RLE to allow safe and Ⓘ transfers.
2. Structured home ambulation program to increase ambulation endurance to 5 min and to improve safety.
3. Gait training on stairs to allow exit from home.
4. Transfer training from a variety of surfaces with emphasis on getting in/out of bed.

Treatment will be 2(/week for 3 weeks. Rehab potential good for meeting goals in 3 weeks and discharge. Plan was reviewed with patient and wife with patient agreeable.

Initial Treatment:
7-12-00   Gait training and transfer training in/out of bed initiated. Pt. ambulated touching R toes only on initial contact. Able to lightly place heel on floor with verbal cues. Pt. required frequent cueing for heel/toe pattern. In/out bed transfers required moderate assist with LEs. Reviewed total hip protocol with pt. and wife; they seemed to understand. Pt. correctly demonstrated home exercises after instructions (see copy in chart), and wife was able to assist pt. with R hip abduction and SLR. Will refer pt. to Joe Jones, PTA, for next 5 visits, and PT will see pt. on 6th visit. Anticipate discharge evaluation at that time.

Signed: Mary Williams, MS, PT, Lic. #123

EXERCISES

7.1. You are Joe Jones, PTA, and you have just made a home visit and treated Mr. X. Review the following notes you took during the treatment session, and write your progress note.

7-17-00

Pt. in good mood, no c/o pain.
Exercises: 10 reps each. Standing at kitchen counter—toe raises, partial knee bends, hip abd, gentle hyperextension, hamstring curls. Supine—SLR with approx. 60–70% assist, bent knee abd.
Sitting—long arc quads.

Amb. in house, good, supervision, 3 point, step-through gait, 1 crutch on L, erect posture, heel/toe pattern. ① up/down stairs in house and porch.

Said able to shower with SBA from wife. Used high stool, sit, swing leg over tub, stand. C/o intense mm spasms after sitting in easy chair. C/o "clink" in hip area with active extension.

Recommend raising chair on platform, notify Dr. if spasms persist/worse, perform extension ex. gently and stop if feels clink again, recommend use 2 crutches if fatigued.

Next visit = 7-25-00

_____

_____

_____

_____

_____

_____

7.2. Use the Guidelines for Critiquing the Progress Note (see p. 139 and identify ways to improve the following progress note:

7-25-00

_____

PT Dx: Decreased ROM & strength RLE interfering with transfers & ambulation safety and endurance.

_____

S: "I saw the doctor yesterday. He thinks everything looks good."

O: Pt. c/o pain when walking outside. Ambulated pt. with one crutch, 3 point heel/toe gait pattern. Instructed on stairs. Pt. states he is bearing about 75% of his wt. on RLE. RLE exercises 10×. Instructed pt. to hold abduction for 3 counts to increase difficulty.

A: Pt. pleased with progress. Progress toward goals 95%. Needs two more visits.

P: Will notify PT about discharge evaluation next week.

—Joe Jones, PTA

_____

_____

_____

_____

_____

_____

7.3. Critique the following progress note:

7-27-00 **PT Dx:** Decreased ROM and strength RLE interfering with transfers and ambulation safety and endurance.

Pt. described discomfort in R hip when leg tires as "hip socket feels thicker." While ambulating with cane during treatment session, pt. reported he didn't feel as steady as with the crutch and the cane is harder on his L wrist. States he continues to have his wife stand by when he is showering. Pt. ① performed his THA exercises supine in bed 10 reps each/heel slides, abduction with powder board, SLR, short arc quads over folded pillow, ankle pumps, isometrics for quads, gluts, hams/RLE exercises standing at kitchen counter per previous note with encouragement to hold abduction 3 counts/reminders to breathe during the exercise. Pt. demonstrated ① bed mobility and sit ↔ stand from elevated easy chair/elevated toilet seat/kitchen chair/bed. Pt. ① ambulated outside 4 min with one crutch, heel/toe, step through, full wt.-bearing gait, demonstrating good balance and erect posture. ① went up/down 3 stairs, no railing. Pt. ambulated with single-end cane in house for first time with min. assist for sense of security and verbal cues, demonstrating slight trunk lean to R (Trendelenburg lurch). Pt./wife encouraged to practice walking short distances in the house with the cane. Progress toward functional outcomes listed in initial eval: #1 met; #2 80%, needs to build endurance to 5-min walk and gain confidence with cane; #3 met. Pt. needs one more visit to work on ambulation and balance with cane and anticipate discharge at that time. Will schedule PT for discharge evaluation.

—Joe Jones, PTA, Lic. #123

_____

_____

_____

_____

_____

_____

7.4. Refer to the initial evaluation for Mr. X with the failed hip prosthesis. The following questions relate to this evaluation.
  a. Read the physical therapy diagnosis identified in the evaluation. List the impairments and the functional limitations.

_____

_____

_____

_____

b. Copy the functional outcomes planned in the evaluation. Circle the action, underline how the outcome will be measured, and draw a line through the time period.

_____

_____

_____

_____

c. Copy the intervention plans from the evaluation. Circle the intervention, underline how the plan will be measured, and draw a line through the frequency and duration. Describe how the impairments will be treated and describe the functional activities.

_____

_____

_____

_____

d. Critique the progress note you wrote in Exercise 7.1 (p. 151).

_____

_____

_____

_____

Practice Exercise 8 ➤   *The following is a physical therapy initial examination/evaluation, followed by related questions.*

LONG-TERM CARE FACILITY: PHYSICAL THERAPY EXAMINATION/EVALUATION

Patient's name: _____   Date of initial evaluation: 8-7-00

Room number: _____   Physician: _____

Date of birth: _____

Diagnosis: Dementia, peripheral vascular disease, atrial fibrillation, heel pressure ulcers bilaterally.

Onset: 7-31-00.

Patient evaluated at bedside. Nursing reported they do two-person lifts to move patient in bed and to transfer to chair. Patient alert but communicated in a confused manner. Pressure ulcers observed on both heels, L greater than R. R wound bed covered with black, thick eschar. Borders detached with red granulation tissue. Significant callous formation around perimeter. No foul odor, minimal drainage. L wound red around edge, significant callous formation around edge. Wound bed covered with blister with dark purple discoloration. Open area in blister/broken blister with minimal drainage, no foul odor.

	R Heel	L Heel
Stage:	Stage III	Stage II
Shape:	Round	Round
Size:	3.9 (horiz) 3 3.4 (vert) cm	Open area 4.3 × 7.2 cm
		Blistered area 6 × 7.3 cm
		Red periphery 11 × 12 cm
Drainage:	Minimum, serous	Minimum, serous

Physical Therapy Diagnosis: Bil. heel pressure ulcers with necrotic tissue and blister interfering with healing, bed mobility, and transfers.

Goals: Debride necrotic tissue in 3 days for clean wound with healthy tissue to enhance healing for eventual assisted bed mobility and assisted pivot transfers.

Intervention Plan: Pulsavac* jet lavage to clean wound and loosen blister and necrotic tissue, followed by debridement of loose skin and necrotic tissue to promote healing, both heels, 1×/day for 3 days.

Initial Treatment: Standard Pulsavac treatment/both heels/bedside/sterile towel under feet with pad underneath. Loose skin from blister debrided on L, healthy tissue under. Eschar trimmed from edges on R. Feet wrapped in sterile towel following, nursing notified; they will dress wounds.

—PT signature, Lic. #xxxxxx

INSTRUCTIONS

Answer the following questions that refer to the initial examination and evaluation of the patient with bilateral pressure ulcers on heels.

8.1. Does the examination contain subjective data? Explain.

_____

_____

_____

8.2. Does the objective data paint a picture of the wounds? Explain.

_____

_____

_____

*Pulsavac III Wound Debridement System, Zimmer Patient Care Division, Dover, OH.

8.3. Is the objective data reproducible? Explain.

_____

_____

_____

8.4. What is (are) the impairment(s)?

_____

_____

_____

8.5. What is (are) the functional limitation(s)?

_____

_____

_____

8.6. What is the purpose of the intervention plan?

_____

_____

_____

8.7. What is the frequency and duration of the intervention plan?

_____

_____

_____

8.8. Copy the goal. *Circle* the action, *underline* the criteria for the goal to be met, and *draw a line through* the time period.

_____

_____

_____

8.9. Assume you are an experienced PTA and have had extra training in wound care. The PT has confidence in your skills to debride and treat these wounds.

    a. Can you duplicate the treatment? Explain.

_____

_____

_____

    b. How will you know when to have the PT do the discharge evaluation/summation of care documentation?

_____

_____

_____

    c. List ways you can document the progress.

_____

_____

_____

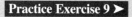 **Practice Exercise 9 ▶**

Many topics about producing quality documentation have been presented in this text. Go back to Chapter 1 and reread the story about the PT's court experience in 1968. Many of the topics in the text are illustrated or suggested in the story. List as many topics as you can.

_____

_____

_____

_____

_____

_____

_____

➤ BIBLIOGRAPHY

American Physical Therapy Association: Guide to Physical Therapist Practice. APTA, Alexandria, VA, July 1999.

American Physical Therapy Association and the Section on Pediatrics: Individualized educational program and individualized family service plan. In Martin, KD (ed.): Physical Therapy Practice in Educational Environments: Policies and Guidelines. APTA, Alexandria, VA, 1990, p 6.1.

Anderson, K, and Anderson, L: Mosby's Pocket Dictionary of Medicine, Nursing, & Allied Health. Mosby, St. Louis, 1990

Baeten, AM, et al: Documenting Physical Therapy: The Reviewer Perspective. Butterworth-Heinemann, Woburn, MA. 1999.

Bernstein, F, et al: Insurance reimbursement and the physical therapist: Documentation for outpatient physical therapy; Guidelines based on California state law. Clin Manage Phys Ther 2:28–33, 1987.

Brown, SR: Physical therapy documentation—Part III. The Pyramid 17:2, 1987.

Cutone, J: One PTA's experience: Team collaboration in the school setting. PT Magazine 3:48, 1994.

Davis, C, and Lippert, L: Facilitators: Reaching agreement about key content areas in PTA curricula. PTA educators colloquium, September 16–17, 1994, Minneapolis. Proceedings to be published by American Physical Therapy Association, Alexandria, VA.

Delitto, A, and Snyder-Mackler, L: The diagnostic process. Examples in orthopedic physical therapy. Phys Ther 3:203, 1995.

Duncan, P: Balance Dysfunction and Motor Control Theory. Workshop notes, April 7–8, 1995, College of St. Scholastica, Duluth, MN.

Esposto, L: Applying functional outcome assessment to Medicare documentation. In Stewart, DL, and Abeln, SH (eds): Documenting Functional Outcomes in Physical Therapy. Mosby, St. Louis, 1993.

Feitelberg, SB (Presenter): A systematic approach to documentation: The basis for successful reimbursement. American Rehabilitation Educational Network (AREN) teleconference, March 19, 1991.

Government Affairs Department: Physical Therapy Practice without Referral: "Direct Access." American Physical Therapy Association, Alexandria, VA, 1992.

Guccione, A: Functional assessment. In O'Sullivan, SB, and Schmitz, JJ (eds): Physical Rehabilitation, Assessment, and Treatment. FA Davis, Philadelphia, 1994.

Hebert, L.: Basics of Medicare documentation for physical therapy. Clinical Management, 1:3, 1981, p 13.

Hill, JR: The Problem-Oriented Approach to Physical Therapy Care. American Physical Therapy Association, Alexandria, VA, 1987.

Jette, AM: Using health-related quality of life measures in physical therapy outcomes research. Phys Ther 8:528, 1993.

Langley, GB, and Sheppeard, H. The visual analogue scale: Its use in pain measurement. Rheumatol Int 5:145, 1985.

Lunning, S (Presenter): Opportunity or chaos? Prepare for the future in physical therapy. Minnesota Chapter American Physical Therapy Association Peer Review Workshop, May 10, 1994, Virginia, MN.

Lupi-Williams, FA: The PTA role & function: An analysis in three parts. Part 1: Education. Clin Manage Phys Ther 3:3, 1983.

McGuire, DB: The measurement of clinical pain. Nurs Res 3:152, 1984.

Melzack, R: The McGill Pain Questionnaire: Major properties and scoring methods. Pain 1:277, 1975.

Moffat, M: Foreward. Journal of Physical Therapy Education 9:35, Fall 1995.

Montgomery, P, and Connolly, B: Motor Control and Physical Therapy: Theoretical Framework, Practical Application, First Edition. Chattanooga Group, Hixson, TN, 1991.

Nagi, SZ: Disability and Rehabilitation. Ohio State University Press, Columbus, 1969.

Ransford, A, et al: The pain drawing as an aid to the psychologic evaluation of patients with low-back pain. Spine 1:127, 1976.

Rogers, J: PTA utilization: The big picture. Clin Manage Phys Ther 11:4, July/August 1991, p 8.

Rose, S: Diagnosis: Defining the term. Phys Ther 69:162, 1989.

Stewart, DL, and Abeln, SH: Documenting Functional Outcomes in Physical Therapy. Mosby, St. Louis, 1993.

Swanson, G: Essentials for the Future of Physical Therapy, Every Therapist's Concern. A Continuing Education Course. Minnesota Chapter American Physical Therapy Association, December 1995, Duluth, MN.

Task Force on Standards for Measurement in Physical Therapy: Standards for tests and measurements in physical therapy practice. Phys Ther 71:589, 1991.

Terminology Task Force of the Acute Care/Hospital Clinical Practice Section of American Physical Therapy Association: Common Terminology, First Draft. Decatur, GA, November 1994.

Thomas, CL (ed): Taber's Cyclopedic Medical Dictionary, Seventeenth Edition. FA Davis, Philadelphia, 1993.

Yaeger, J: Effective listening techniques. Notes from Mgt 503, Oral Communication. Masters in Management Program. College of St. Scholastica, Duluth, MN, 1990.

➤ GLOSSARY

Accountable: Responsible, capable of explaining oneself.

Accredit: To supply with credentials or authority.

Accreditation: Granting of approval to an institution by an official review board after the institution has met specific requirements.

Adhesive capsulitis: A condition characterized by adhesions and shortening or tightening of the connective tissue sleeve that encases a joint.

Ambulate: To walk about.

American Physical Therapy Association: Professional organization representing the physical therapy profession, the occupation consisting of professionals and technicians trained to provide the medical rehabilitative service of physical therapy.

Antalgic: Painful or indicating the presence of pain.

Anterior capsule: Front portion of the joint connective tissue sleeve.

Assessment: Measurement, quantification, or placement of a value or label on something; assessment is often confused with evaluation; an assessment results from the act of assessing.*

Ataxia: Condition characterized by impaired ability to coordinate movement. Ataxic gait is a staggering, uncoordinated walk.

Audit: Examination of records to check accuracy and compliance with professional standards.

Authenticate: To verify, to prove, to establish as worthy of belief.

Autonomy: Independence, ability to self-govern.

Biomechanics: Study of mechanical laws and their application to living organisms, especially the human body.

Circumduct: To move the joint in a circular manner.

Clinical decision: Determination that relates to direct patient care, indirect patient care, acceptance of patients for treatment, and whether patients should be referred to other practitioners.† A diagnosis that leads a therapist to take an action is a form of a clinical decision; clinical decisions result in actions; when direct supporting evidence for clinical decisions is lacking, such decisions are based on clinical opinions.

Collaborate: To work together, to cooperate.

Concentric contraction: Muscle contraction that moves the muscle from a resting, lengthened position to a shortened position; a muscle contraction in which the insertion and origin move closer together.

Continuum: A continuous extent, succession, or whole.

Coordination: Muscle action of the appropriate intensity, timing, and sequencing to produce a smooth, controlled, purposeful movement.

Criteria: Requirements, standards, rules.

Data: Information, especially information organized for analysis or used as the basis for a decision.

Direct access: Legislation that enables the consumer to enter the medical care system by going directly to a PT. The patient needing physical therapy treatment does not need to be referred to a PT by a physician.

Disability: The inability to engage in age-specific, gender-related, and sex-specific roles in a particular social context and physical environment.‡

Discharge evaluation: Made only by a PT on termination of treatment by the PT. It contains recommendations and decisions about future treatment.

Discharge summary: A document that may be written by the PTA stating the treatments provided and the status of the patient at time of discharge. If this document contains recommendations or decisions about future treatment, it is considered an evaluation and must be written by the PT.

Documentation: Written information supplying proof, a written record, supporting references.

Duration: Period of time in which something persists or exists.

Eccentric contraction: A muscle contraction that moves the muscle from a shortened position to its lengthened or resting position; muscle contraction in which the insertion and origin move away from each other.

Edema: Swelling; accumulation of fluid in the tissues.

Efficacy: Effectiveness, ability to achieve results.

Episode of care: All physical therapy services that are (1) provided by a physical therapist or under the direction and supervision of a physical therapist, (2) provided in an unbroken sequence, and (3) related to the physical therapy interventions for a given condition or problem or related to a request from the patient/client, family, or other health care provider.‡

Evaluation: Judgment based on a measurement; often confused with assessment and examination; evaluations are judgments of the value or worth of something. A dynamic process in which the physical therapist makes clinical judgments based on data gathered during the examination.‡

Examination: Test or a group of tests used for the purpose of obtaining measurements or data.* The process of obtaining a history, performing relevant systems reviews, and selecting and administering specific tests and measurements.‡

Extension: Movement of a joint in which the angle between the two adjoining bones increases.

Facilitate: To enhance or help an action or function.

Femur: Thigh bone.

Flexion: Movement of a joint in which the angle between the two adjoining bones decreases.

Fractured: Broken. Typically refers to broken bones.

Frequency: Number of times something occurs, number of repetitions, number of treatment sessions.

Functional limitation: Restriction of the ability to perform a physical action, activity, or task in an efficient, typically expected, or competent manner.‡

Gait: Walking pattern.

Girth: Distance around something, circumference.

Goniometry: Procedure for measuring the range of motion angles of a joint.

Hamstrings: Common name for the group of three muscles located on the posterior thigh.

Hip extensors: Common name for the group of muscles that produce extension motion of the hip joint.

Hypertonus: Excessive muscle tone or prolonged muscle contraction.

Impairment: A loss or abnormality of physiologic, psychologic, or anatomic structure or function.‡

Incident: Distinct occurrence; an event inconsistent with usual routine or treatment procedure; an accident.

Incident report: Documentation required when an unusual event occurs in a clinic or medical facility.

Individual educational program: Written statement outlining the goals and objectives for the services provided to meet a physically disabled child's educational needs.

Informed consent: Permission or agreement for medical treatment based on knowledge of all the information about the treatment.

Initial and mid swing: Portions of the walking pattern when the heel and then the toes leave the ground and the leg swings to the point where the hip is at 0° flexion or extension.

Internship: Period of time during which a medical professional in training provides clinical care under supervision.

Intervention: The purposeful and skilled interaction of the physical therapist with the patient/client and, when appropriate, with other individuals involved in care, using various methods and techniques to produce changes in the condition.‡

Joint Commission on Accreditation of Healthcare Organizations: Agency with the responsibility to ensure that hospitals and medical centers follow federal and state regulations and meet the standards necessary for the provision of safe and appropriate health care.

Laceration: Torn, jagged wound.

Lag: To fall behind, not keep up, develop slowly, weaken, or slacken.

Lower extremity: Area that includes the thigh, lower leg, and foot.

Medicaid: Federally funded, state-administered health insurance for eligible individuals with low income who are too young to qualify for Medicare.

Medical diagnosis: Identification of a systemic disease or disorder based on the findings from a physician's examination and diagnostic test.

Medicare: Federally funded national health insurance for certain persons older than 65.

Mobilization techniques: Manual techniques or procedures used by physical therapy professionals to increase the range of motion of a joint.

Modality: Method of therapy or treatment procedure.

Muscle spasms: Persistent, involuntary contractions of a muscle or certain groups of muscle fibers within the muscle.

Negligence: State of being extremely careless or lacking in concern.

Neuromusculoskeletal: Pertaining to the nervous system, the muscular system, and the skeletal system.

Occupational therapist: Trained health care professional who provides occupational therapy.

Occupational therapy assistant: Trained health-care technician who provides occupational therapy under the supervision of an occupational therapist.

Orthopedics: Branch of medicine devoted to the study and treatment of the skeletal system and its joints, muscles, and associated structures.

Palpable: Able to be felt or touched.

Parameters: Limits or boundaries; a value or constant used to describe or measure a set of data representing a physiologic function or system.

Paraparesis: Partial paralysis or extreme weakness.

Pathokinesiologic: Pertaining to the study of movements relating to a given disorder.

Pathologic: Pertaining to a condition that is caused by or involves a disease.

Pathology: Study of the characteristics, causes, and effects of disease.

Physical therapist assistant: A technically educated health care provider who assists the physical therapist in the provision of physical therapy. The physical therapist assistant, under the direction and supervision of the physical therapist, is the only paraprofessional who provides physical therapy interventions. The physical therapist assistant is a graduate of a physical therapist assistant associated degree program accredited by the Commission on Accreditation in Physical Therapy (CAPTE).‡

Physical therapy: The treatment of impairments and functional limitations by physical means such as exercise, education and training, heat, light, electricity, water, cold, ultrasound, massage, and manual therapy to improve or restore the patient's ability to function in his or her environment. Physical therapy is provided by trained persons who have graduated from accredited physical therapy and physical therapist assistant schools.

Physical Therapy Practice Act: Legislation in each state that defines and regulates the practice or provision of physical therapy services.

Physical therapy problem: Identification of the neuromusculoskeletal dysfunction and resulting functional limitation that is treatable by physical therapy.

Physician assistants: Trained technicians performing medical care under the supervision of a physician.

Problem-oriented: Based on or directed toward the problem, as in the medical record organized around the identification of the medical problems.

Prone: Horizontal and face-down position.

Psoriasis: A common, chronic, inheritable skin disorder characterized by circumscribed red patches covered by thick, dry, silvery, adherent scales.

Quadriparesis: Partial paralysis or extreme weakness of arms, legs, and trunk resulting from injury to spinal nerves in the cervical spine.

Quality assurance: Title of the department, usually in health care facilities, that reviews medical charts to identify when regulations and standards are not being met or when unsafe or inappropriate medical care is provided.

Quality assurance committee: Group that performs chart reviews.

Rehabilitation facilities: Clinics or institutions that provide rehabilitation services such as physical therapy, occupational therapy, speech pathology, psychologic services, social services, orthotics and prosthetics, and patient and family education.

Reimbursement: Payment for services.

Release-of-information form: Document that the patient signs to give permission for the person(s) named in the document to receive information about the patient's medical condition and treatment.

Reliable: Dependable, reproducible.

Retrospective: Looking back on, contemplating, or directed to the past.

Rule of confidentiality: A principle that information about patients should not be revealed to anyone not authorized to receive the information.

Signs: Characteristics or indications of disease or dysfunction determined by objective tests, measurements, or observations.

Source-oriented: Organized around the source of the information, as in the medical record organized according to the various disciplines providing and documenting the care.

Speech pathologist: Trained professional who diagnoses and treats abnormalities of speech.

Status quo: No change in a specified state or condition.

Symptoms: Subjective characteristics or indications of disease or dysfunction as perceived by the patient.

Systemic: Pertaining to the whole body.

Tactile: Pertaining to the sense of touch.

Vital signs: Measurements of pulse rate, respiration rate, body temperature, and blood pressure.

Workers' compensation: State- and business-funded health insurance that manages and funds medical care for persons injured on the job.

---

*Task Force on Standards for Measurement in Physical Therapy: Standards for tests and measurement in physical therapy practice. Phys Ther 71:589, 1991.

†This definition is modified from that presented by Charles Magistro at a conference on Clinical Decision Making held under APTA auspices in October 1988 in Lake of the Ozarks, MO.

‡American Physical Therapy Association: Guide to Physical Therapist Practice. APTA, Alexandria, VA. Appendix 1, July 1999.

Abbreviations

↔	to/from	DOB	date of birth
↑	increase	Dx	diagnosis
↓	decrease	Elec.	electrical
//	parallel	ER	emergency room, external rotation
&	and		
1X	one time, one person	E-stim	electrical stimulation
2o	secondary to	Ev, ev	eversion
ā	before	Eval	evaluation
A	assessment	ex.	exercise
abd/add	abduction/adduction	ext.	extension
ADL	activities of daily living	F	female, fair muscle strength grade
AFO	ankle foot orthosis		
AM, a.m.	morning	FAROM	functional active range of motion
amb.	ambulation		
appts	appointments	FES	functional electrical stimulation
APTA	American Physical Therapy Association		
		flex	flexion
AAROM	active assistive range of motion	FOR	functional outcome report
		ft	foot, feet
AROM	active range of motion	F/U	follow up
assist	assistance	FWB	full weight bearing
B	bilateral, both	FWW, fw/w	front wheeled walker
bid	twice a day	Fx	fracture(d)
bil.	bilateral	G	good muscle strength grade
BLE	both lower extremities	gastrocs	gastrocnemius muscles
BP	blood pressure	gluts	gluteals
BPM	beats per minute	GMT	gross muscle test
c̄	with	Gt.	gait
CARF	Commission on Accreditation of Rehabilitation Facilities	hams	hamstrings
		HEP	home exercise program
CCs	chief complaints	HCFA	Health Care Financing Administration
cm	centimeter(s)		
c/o	complains of, complaint(s) of	HHA	home health aide
coord	coordination	HNP	herniated nucleus pulposus
CP	compression pump	HP	hot pack
CPM	continuous passive motion machine	hr	hour
		HS	hamstring(s)
CVA	cerebral vascular accident	Hx	history
CW	continuous wave	Ⓘ	independent(ly)
D₁, D₂	diagonal 1, diagonal 2	ICIDH	International Classification of Impairments, Disabilities, and Handicaps
d/c	discharged, discontinued		
DEP	data, evaluation, performance goals		
		ICIDH-2	International Classification of Functioning and Disability
DF	dorsiflexion		
DJD	degenerative joint disease	ICP	intermittent compression pump
DNR	do not recusitate		

IEP	individual education program	PT	physical therapist
int.	internal	PTA	physical therapist assistant
IV	inversion	PWB	partial weight bearing
JCAHO	Joint Commission on Accreditation of Healthcare Organizations	quads	quadriceps
		R	right
		RA	rheumatoid arthritis
L	left	re:	regarding
L5	5th lumbar vertebra	re-ed	re-education
LAQ	long arc quadriceps	reps	repetitions
lat.	lateral	ret.	return
lb	pound	RLE	right lower extremity
LBP	low back pain	r/o	rule out
LE	lower extremities	ROM	range of motion
Lic	license	rot.	rotation
LLE	left lower extremity	RUE	right upper extremity
LOB	loss of balance	S	subjective data, status
LUE	left upper extremity	SAQ	short arc quadriceps
M	male	SBA	standby assist
max.	maximum	SCI	spinal cord injury
MD	Medical Doctor	SEC	single-end cane
mech	mechanical	sec	second(s)
MH	moist heat	SLR	straight leg raise
MHz	MegaHertz	SOAP	subjective, objective, assessment, plan
min	minutes		
min.	minimal, minimum	SOMR	source-oriented medical record
mmHg	millimeters of mercury		
mm(s)	muscle(s)	SPTA	student physical therapist assistant; physical therapist assistant student
MMT	manual muscle test		
mod.	moderate		
N/A	not able	STG	short-term goal
neg.	negative	str.	strength
noc.	night	strep	Streptococcus
NWB	non–weight-bearing	SWD	shortwave diathermy
O	objective data	Sx	symptoms
occ	occasional	TDD	tentative discharge data
OOB	out of bed	TDP	tentative discharge plan
OP	outpatient	T.E.D.s	antiembolism stockings
OT	occupational therapist	temp.	temperature
p̄	after	TFs	transfers
P	poor muscle grade strength, Plan	THA	total hip arthroplasty
		ther. ex.	therapeutic exercise
per	by	tid	three times a day
PF	plantarflexion	TKA	total knee arthroplasty
PM, p.m.	afternoon	TKE	terminal knee extension
POC	plan of care	TMJ	temporomandibular joint
POMR	problem-oriented medical record	trng.	training
		TTWB	toe touch weight bearing
pps	pulses per second	TWB	touch weight bearing
Pr	problem	tx	treatment
PRE	progressive resistive exercise	UE	upper extremity
PRN, PRN	as needed	UED1	upper extremity diagonal 1
PROM	passive range of motion	US	ultrasound
PSP	problem, status, plan	w/	with
PSPG	problem, status, plan, goals	WBAT	weight bearing as tolerated
pt.	patient	WC, w/c	wheelchair

w/cm^2	watts per square centimeter	wt.	weight
WFL	within functional limits	X	times
WHO	World Health Organization	yr	year
wlp	whirlpool	YO	year(s) old
w/o	without	YOM	year old male
WNL	within normal limits		

APPENDIX B

Documenting Interventions

SUGGESTED INTERVENTION DOCUMENTATION STYLE

Documenting interventions thoroughly enough so they can be reproduced by another PTA or PT while still keeping the progress note as brief as possible is not easy. The following is a method for providing the appropriate information in a concise format. In this "formula" style for documenting interventions, the information is placed in a continuous line separated by slashes. A list of information that should be included for the intervention to be reproducible is provided on page 78–79. The information is documented as illustrated here but does not have to be placed in this order. Type of intervention/dosage or intensity/treatment area/time/patient position/frequency/purpose.

Examples

Direct contact US/3 MHz/mild heat at (0.5 w/cm^2)/right TMJ/sitting/5 min/to decrease inflammation.

Direct contact US/1 MHz/(1w/cm^2)/7 min/left middle trapezius & rhomboid/prone/to relax spasm.

Direct contact US/1 MHz/(1.5 w/cm^2)/5 min/L shoulder, anterior capsule/sitting/to prepare for stretching.

Induction SWD/large pad/dose III/vigorous heat/L1 to S2/prone/20 min to prepare for stretching.

Intermittent cervical traction/Saunders halter/supine/15 lb/30 sec on, 10 sec off/20 min/to stretch C1–C4 cervical extensors.

Immersion US/1 MHz/right deltoid ligament/sitting/(2 w/cm^2)/10 min/to prepare for stretching

Static pelvic traction/L4–L5/prone/100 lb/10 min max. or until pain centralizes/to reduce disc bulge.

Ice massage/standard procedure/to numbing response/R wrist extensors' tendons at origin/sitting, shoulder abducted 90°, elbow flexed 90° on pillow/after exercise/to minimize inflammatory response.

Hot packs/R biceps femoris muscle belly/12 towel layers/prone/20 min/to increase circulation for healing.

Foot whirlpool/110°/decubitus on L lateral malleolus/sitting in wheelchair/for mechanical debridement/20 min.

ICP/50 lb/30 sec on, 10 sec off/RUE/elevated 45°/supine/3 hr/to decrease edema.

FES/L anterior tibialis/monopolar/one channel, three leads/two 2-inch square electrodes/origin & insertion/nontreatment electrode under R thigh/30 pps/15 min/motor response/pt. semi-sitting/for muscle re-education and AAROM.

➤ APPENDIX C

Dictation Guidelines

In some clinical facilities you will dictate your progress notes instead of writing them. You will dictate or speak into a recording device (such as a small tape recorder or into a telephone), and a medical transcriptionist will listen to the tape and type your note. The typed note will be returned to you to proof read and sign. When learning to dictate progress notes, take the time to write the note first on scrap paper. Then you can read it out loud into the recorder. After you become accustomed to the dictation procedure, you will be able to compose the note and dictate it simultaneously.

GUIDELINES FOR CLEAR DICTATION

1. Keep in mind that each facility will have guidelines for PTAs. In one clinic, the transcriptionist may be so skilled in typing physical therapy documentation that you will do little more than dictate the content. A medical transcriptionist typically has been trained at a 2-year technical college or community college program. The trained transcriptionist is knowledgeable in medical terminology and punctuation. Another clinic may require that you give specific instructions to the transcriptionist and dictate punctuation. In either case, follow these guidelines for clear dictation.
2. Use proper sentence structure and punctuation, although you can eliminate some wording to keep the note brief.
3. Introduce your dictation by telling the transcriptionist *who you are,* that this is a *progress note,* the *name of your patient,* and the *date of treatment.*
4. Spell out any foreign or unusual names of muscles, treatment techniques, or diagnoses. Clarify <u>ab</u>duct and <u>ad</u>duct by spelling out the word.
5. Tell the transcriptionist when you are starting or finishing a note on a particular patient or date, particularly if you are dictating more than one note on a tape.
6. Give your full legal name with your proper abbreviated title (SPTA or PTA) at the end of the dictation.
7. Do not sniff, cough, or chew gum while dictating into the dictaphone.
8. Speak clearly and slowly. Do not mumble.
9. Do not say "uhhh." If you need to collect your thoughts, turn off the tape.

In clinics that require you to give specific instructions to the transcriptionist, follow these additional guidelines:

1. State "operator" just before your instructions to alert the transcriptionist that instructions are to follow, not content.
2. Tell the transcriptionist what letters you want capitalized. However, you can assume the transcriptionist will automatically capitalize the first letter of each sentence. For example: You might say, "Patient's (operator: all in caps) ROM (operator: end of caps) is 0–90 degrees for left knee flexion."
3. Tell the transcriptionist when you are moving to a new heading. For example: "(operator: new heading, all in caps) objective" will come back to you typed "OBJECTIVE."
4. Be aware that you may need to dictate some of the punctuation. For example: You want your note to read, "<u>T</u>ransfers:①out recliner, on/off toilet, bed after four tries." Your dictation should sound like this: "(Operator: underline capital T) transfers colon independent out recliner comma on slash off toilet comma bed after four tries period."

Answers to Review Exercises

CHAPTER 1   Review exercises are on page 11.

1. If there is no documentation that medical care was provided, it is assumed the care did not occur or was not given.

2. First, physicians prescribed the therapy and told the PT exactly what treatments to do. Later, the prescription just referred the patient to the PT with a diagnosis, and the PT could evaluate and decide what treatments were appropriate. Finally, direct access legislation allows the PT to see, evaluate, and treat a patient without the patient first going to a physician for referral.

3. First, the PT was a technician, following the exact orders of the physician. Later, the PT added evaluation skills and made decisions about treatment plans, and the PTA carried out the plans under PT supervision. Now the PT consults, evaluates, and recognizes when to refer a patient to a physician or another more appropriate health-care provider. The PTA continues to carry out the treatment plan but does not require on-site supervision and is part of the PT–PTA team.

4. *Direct access* means a person can see a PT without obtaining a physician's referral. The first medical professional seeing the patient may be a PT, and the PT may refer the patient to another appropriate health-care provider. Thus a person can access the health-care system through physical therapy.

5. Limited funding for the provision of health care and the need for providers to compete for the funds. The PT and PTA should be responsible for good documentation that demonstrates accountability and quality of care.

6. The medical record is (1) a record of the quality of the medical care provided to the patient, (2) a legal document providing evidence of the care, and (3) the method by which third-party payers determine the value of the care provided and reimbursement for that care.

7. The record is audited to ensure that the standards and criteria for quality care and documentation are followed.

8. The federal government, state government, accrediting agencies, professional agencies, and the individual health facility.

9. Following the policies and procedures where you work ensures that your documentation will meet the necessary standards or criteria.

CHAPTER 2   Review exercises are on page 22.

1. a. Data: The subjective and objective information that is gathered about the patient and why he or she is seeking medical treatment.

   b. Problems: The problems that require medical treatment as determined by interpretation of the data.

   c. Treatment plan: The description of the treatment appropriate for the problems.

   d. Purpose, goals, desired outcomes: Statements describing what the treatment should accomplish.

   e. Treatment procedures administered: A record of the treatments provided through progress notes, flow charts, checklists, or brief statements.

f. Results or effectiveness of the treatment: Statements as to whether the treatment accomplished its intended purpose or goal.

2. Subjective data comprise the information provided by the patient or a representative of the patient. These data are what the patient tells the medical person. Objective data comprise the information gathered by a health-care provider through tests, measurements, observations, and examinations. This information can be reproduced by another health-care provider with the same training.

3. *Symptoms* are the feelings, experiences, or complaints the patient describes that cause the patient to seek medical attention. The objective information gathered from tests, measurements, and observations are the *signs* of the disease or pathology.

4. The *medical diagnosis* is a systemic disease or disorder determined by the physician through physical examination and diagnostic tests. The *physical therapy diagnosis* is the identification of one or more anatomical abnormalities or dysfunctions resulting in one or more functional limitations or difficulties causing the patient to seek physical therapy. The physical therapy diagnosis can be the medical diagnosis, or a patient may have both a medical diagnosis and a PT diagnosis.

5. The PT is responsible for writing all examinations and evaluations, goals and outcomes, and intervention plans for the patient. Both the PT and the PTA write progress notes.

6. The three types of examinations/evaluations are the initial examination, interim or reexaminations and reevaluations, and the discharge examination or summation of care. The PTA may assist the PT with the examination by taking notes, performing and recording the results of tests or measurements in accordance with the PTA's training, and establishing a rapport with the patient. The PTA plans the treatment sessions based on the PT's intervention plan, objectives, and goals and functional outcomes.

7. A *discharge evaluation* summarizes the treatment the patient received, discusses the results, identifies whether the treatment was effective, and makes recommendations or states what is planned for the patient after discharge. This evaluation must be documented by a PT. A PTA is permitted to write a *discharge summary* that simply lists the interventions provided and describes the patient's status at discharge time. In the discharge summary, the PTA is not to make recommendations or decisions regarding the patient's treatment following discharge. The final note in the PT chart about the patient must be written by the PT.

CHAPTER 3   Review exercises are on page 43.

1. SOMR is the abbreviation for source-oriented medical record. The SOMR is organized into sections according to the disciplines or medical services providing the information. There is a physicians' information section, a nursing section, a physical therapy section, a laboratory test results section, and so on. POMR is the abbreviation for problem-oriented medical record. The POMR is organized into sections according to the information or documentation content, and the content focuses on the problems being treated. The sections consist of the data, problems, treatment plans, progress notes, and discharge notes. Each discipline writes its information in the appropriate section. For example, physical therapy notes and nursing notes would be together in the progress note section, addressing the problem being treated.

2. **S** stands for subjective, and contains information told to the therapist by the patient or someone representing the patient.
   O stands for objective, and contains information gathered from tests, measurements, and observations that can be reproduced by someone else with the same training.
   A stands for assessment, and contains statements that interpret the subjective and objective data. Treatment goals, treatment effectiveness, and outcome are recorded here.
   P stands for plan, and states the treatment plan or what will happen in the next treatment session.

3. PSPG, DEP, and FOR are other models for organizing evaluation and progress note content. PSPG stands for problem, status, plan, and goals. DEP stands for data, evaluation, and performance goals. FOR is the abbreviation for functional outcome report.

4. The PTA can adapt to any organization model by logically sequencing the progress note information in a problem-solving manner. First, identify the problem about which the note is written. Next, report the data gathered during treatment and interpret these data by showing how the information relates to the treatment objectives and functional goals established in the PT's initial evaluation. Finally, report what is planned for the next session. The PTA can easily organize this information into any format.

5. Checklists, flow charts, fill-in-the-blank forms: Typically used in hospitals, long-term care facilities, and rehabilitation centers.
   Narrative or outlined notes, dictated and typed or handwritten: Used in all facilities and can be combined with checklists, flow charts, and other formats.
   Letter: Commonly used by private-practice facilities to communicate with the physician about the patient's treatment progress.
   Individualized educational program: Used in the schools when a physically disabled child requires specialized services such as physical therapy to assist in his or her education.
   Cardex: Used by some facilities to keep up-to-date treatment plans on cards kept within the physical therapy department. These are used by the treating therapists for quick references and are not part of the patient's medical record.
   Medicare standardized forms: Used by health-care personnel to document information when treating patients who have Medicare insurance. These required forms are common in long-term care facilities, rehabilitation centers, home-health-care agencies, and hospitals.

6. The PTA can provide and record only the information that describes the status of the patient and a summary of the interventions that were provided. However, the PTA should not complete the form because it is intended to be an evaluation.

7. The PTA should always follow the facility's documentation policies, procedures, and format.

CHAPTER 4   Review exercises are on page 56.

1. The progress note is the record of the treatment procedures administered. It is written proof that the PT's intervention plan was carried out and it documents the effectiveness of the interventions. Both PTs and PTAs write progress notes, but the PTA's main documentation responsiblity is writing the progress note. Progress notes are written daily for acute care patients and weekly or less often for patients receiving treatment for chronic conditions. Frequency depends on the facility's procedures.

2. Progress notes can be written in SOAP outline; in paragraph style narration; in a combination of checklists, flow sheets, and narrative; on computer software forms; dictated and typed or handwritten; or in formats (e.g., DEP, FOR, PSPG) according to the facility's preference.

3. **Be accurate:** Information about the patient's medical care must be thorough and accurate in case it must be recalled later in court or if questions arise.
   Be brief: Notes must be relevant to the problem being treated and must be thorough, but they should be short so they can be read quickly. Be concise and to the point; do not use excess words.
   Be clear: Everyone who reads the note must be able to understand its meaning. Handwritten notes must be legible, and punctuation, grammar, and spelling must be correct.
   Date and sign all entries: It must be clear when the note was written and who wrote it for reference later if questions arise.

Use black ink: Black ink is most commonly used, but some clinics may prefer to use another color to distinguish the original document from a copy. The document should be clear when photocopied.

Do not allow opportunity for the record to be changed or falsified: The note must be accurate, so you should not leave spaces where information could be inserted and should not use an erasable pen that would enable your information to be changed. Do not erase errors, but instead draw a line through the mistake and date and initial above it so that it is clear who made the change.

Be timely when documenting: The note is more accurate if it is written as soon as possible after the patient's treatment because the information will be fresh in the PTA's mind.

4. Abbreviations are not recommended because not everyone reading the note may know the meaning of the abbreviation. Many reading the note will not want to take the time to look up the meaning of abbreviations. Some may misinterpret the meaning (an abbreviation may have many meanings). Misinterpreting an abbreviation can cause harm to a patient or delay treatment.

5. Many health-care providers other than physical therapy–trained providers use some of the same treatment techniques that are used by PTs and PTAs. Putting the license or registration number after the signature identifies those treatments that were provided by physical therapy-trained personnel. This will help when medical records are researched to determine frequency of use and effectiveness of the treatment techniques.

CHAPTER 5 Review exercises are on page 69.

1. Subjective data consist of information that the patient, a family member, or representative of the patient tells the PT or PTA, and must be relevant to the problem or treatment.

2. Relevant subjective data consist of information that can influence the treatment or goal planning, prove intervention effectiveness or ineffectiveness, or describe a change in the patient's condition. Relevant information consists of the patient's medical history, environment and lifestyle, emotions and attitudes, goals or functional outcomes, unusual events, chief complaints, response to treatment, level of functioning, and pain.

3. Subjective data content can be grouped according to the categories of relevant information listed in Question 2. Organizing the content into these categories makes reading and understanding the information easier than when the content is randomly organized and seems to ramble.

4. Use verbs that inform the reader that the information is being provided by the patient and that the patient is telling the therapist.
   Quote the patient to make the meaning clearer.
   Indicate which information comes from the patient and which information is provided by someone else.
   Remember that any information about pain is subjective data.

5. Pain information is always included in the subjective data content because the patient is perceiving the pain, interpreting the sensation, and reporting or describing it to the therapist.

6. Students often write too much subjective information that is irrelevant to the problem or treatment. Students often make the mistake of failing to include pain information in the subjective data content.

CHAPTER 6 Review exercises are on page 83.

1. Objective data must consist of information that can be reproduced or observed by someone else with the same training.

2. Results of measurements and tests.
   Description of the patient's function.
   Description of the interventions provided.
   Objective observations made by the PTA.

3. Documentation of the results of tests and measurements must be consistent with the method of documentation in the PT's initial evaluation. What is being tested or measured, the position of the patient, the starting and ending points, and the points of measurements, as appropriate, must be clearly written.

4. In describing the patient's function, the PTA should paint a picture of the patient performing the activity. The description should include the activity; type of equipment or assistive devices used; speed, time, or distance; number of repetitions; amount of weight; type of gait pattern; amount of assistance needed and why; the environment; and the quality of the patient's movement.

5. To be reproducible, the treatment description should give the type of intervention; specific machine or piece of equipment, if appropriate; dosage, time, and frequency; parameters or settings; position of patient; target tissue or treatment area; physiologic response desired, if appropriate; and purpose of the intervention.

6. Students commonly make two major mistakes when documenting objective data: (1) writing about what they did rather than discussing what the patient did, and (2) rambling or failing to organize the information into topics.

CHAPTER 7   Review exercises are on page 103.

1. The interpretation of the data in the progress note is the most important content to most readers because it informs the reader whether the treatment is effective and whether the patient is making progress. This is what the insurance representative, physician, lawyer, and supervising PT want to know.

2. *Expected functional outcome* is the expected elimination of or decrease in severity of the patient's functional limitation. The *anticipated goal,* written as a series of steps or desired functional ability broken down into tasks, designates the change in impairment needed for the patient's functional improvement.

3. The action of the function or goal.
   Criteria that can be measured that determines when the outcome/goal is met.
   A time period in which the goal or outcome should be accomplished.

4. The PTA may not determine or write the functional outcomes or goals of the physical therapy treatment. The PTA may confer with the PT and assist with the planning. The PTA may document progress toward and accomplishment of the outcomes and goals with evidence contained in the data in the progress note.

5. Change in the severity of the impairment or functional limitation.
   Progress toward accomplishment of the goals or outcomes.
   Lack of progress or intervention ineffectiveness with recommendations.
   Inconsistencies in the subjective and objective data.

6. Impairment changes are documented by repeating tests and measurements or observations as they were performed and documented in the initial evaluation and comparing the results.
   Progress or lack of progress toward goals is documented (1) by renaming the outcomes or goals, or referring to their numbers as listed in the initial evaluation; and (2) by stating how much progress has been made (or not made) toward accomplishing those specific goals.
   Subjective and objective data should refer to tests, measurements, and functional activities described in the initial evaluation. The inconsistencies should relate to this same information, not to information that is not discussed in the initial evaluation.

7. Making generalized statements such as "pt. tolerated treatment well" and not relating statement to specific information in the data.

Making statements about information that is not mentioned in the data portion of the note.

Talking about new information.

Forgetting to talk about the patient's progress toward improving the functional limitation that brought the patient to physical therapy. Forgetting to talk about the goals or outcomes listed in the initial evaluation.

CHAPTER 8   Review exercises are on page 117.

1. The plan section of the PT's initial evaluation lists the interventions planned to accomplish the goals or outcomes. It describes what will be done to decrease the severity of the impairment and improve the patient's functional abilities. Each intervention listed has an objective or statement as to its purpose. The plan indicates the frequency of treatment and a time period within which the treatment will be given (duration). The interim evaluation contains changes or modifications of the intervention plan, and the discharge evaluation discusses the intervention or follow-up activities needed in the future after discharge.

2. The PTA may not design or modify the intervention plan. The PTA may assist the PT, provide relevant information, and make suggestions.

3. The content of the plan section of the progress note describes what will happen between the time the note was written and the next treatment session, or what will happen at the next session. This section may report the number of remaining treatment sessions the patient is expected to complete. The plan content should include statements about working with the PT.

4. The plan statements provide evidence of PT–PTA teamwork by discussing intentions to consult with the PT, notify the PT, or make recommendations to the PT.

CHAPTER 9   Review exercises are on page 126.

1. Other documentation responsibilities include: documenting telephone conversations, such as referrals and requests for information about the patient's condition.

Documenting the patient's refusal of treatment.

Completing an incident report.

2. The rule of confidentiality is the ethical principle that all information about the patient, such as the treatment and the patient's condition, is private. Only the persons providing that medical care are to have access to the information; anyone else must have permission from the patient to receive the information.

3. Give information about the client only to the persons for whom the client has signed a release-of-information form.

Keep the client's medical record in a location where unauthorized people cannot read it.

Discuss the patient in private and only with persons authorized to have access to the information.

4. The release-of-information form is signed by the patient to authorize a person to receive medical information about the patient. This form protects the confidentiality of the patient by ensuring that the information goes only to those persons whom the patient agrees should know the information.

5. Name of the person referring.

Name of the person calling in the referral, if different from the person doing the referring.

Name of the PTA taking the call.

Name, address, and pertinent information about the client.

Details of the referral.

Date of the call.

Statement that the referral will be mailed to the caller for signature.

Statement that the PT will be notified.

6. If questions arise regarding any aspect of the referral, the persons involved in the telephone conversation can be contacted easily for clarification.

7. First determine why the patient is refusing treatment. Then explore with the patient alternatives or ideas that will satisfy the patient's concerns and allow the treatment to be provided. Explain the consequences of not receiving treatment. If the reason for refusal is valid or the patient persists in refusing, recognize the right of the patient to refuse, document this, and notify the PT.

8. Place a statement in the chart that the patient refused treatment; give the reason, report what the PTA did to encourage treatment, and state that the PT will be or was notified. This statement is placed in lieu of a progress note.

9. An *incident* is anything happening to the patient, an employee, or a visitor that is unusual, out of the ordinary, not part of routine or procedure, or inconsistent with treatment procedures; an accident or a situation that could cause an accident.

10. Name and address of the person involved in the incident, and other pertinent information.
    Date of the incident.
    Name and address of the eyewitness writing the incident report.
    Names and addresses of other eyewitnesses.
    Description and identification of equipment involved.
    Objective, factual description of the incident.
    Description of the action taken at the time of the incident.
    Description of the status or condition of the person involved before and after the incident.
    Description of the environmental conditions before and after the incident.

11. An incident report identifies situations that pose a danger to patients, employees, and visitors. Facilities have risk-management procedures for correcting these situations to maintain a safe environment for everyone. The incident report policy requires a procedure for the provision of immediate medical care or action when an incident occurs. The report provides an objective record of the details if needed in the event of a litigation.

12. The incident report is kept in a separate file because it is confidential hospital information. The incident is documented in the patient's chart, but no mention is made in the patient's medical record that an incident report has been completed.

Answers to Practice Exercises

CHAPTER 2	Practice exercises begin on page 23.

Practice Exercise 1 ➤
The medical problem is fractured right femur.
The abnormality or dysfunction of the musculoskeletal system is decreased strength in quadriceps.
The functional limitation is the inability to transfer independently in and out of bed or chair.

Practice Exercise 2 ➤
The medical diagnosis is cerebral vascular accident.
The abnormality or dysfunction of the neuromuscular system (impairment) is weakness and extensor hypertonus in the left lower extremity.
The functional limitation is the inability to climb stairs independently.

Practice Exercise 3 ➤
The medical diagnosis is incomplete spinal cord injury.
The impairment is lower-extremity paraparesis.
The functional limitation is the inability to stand.

Practice Exercise 4 ➤

   PT   Initial examination and evaluation

   PTA   Progress notes

   PTA   Measurements results

   PT   Reexamination and reevaluation

   PT   Change in treatment plan

   PTA   Discharge summary with no interpretation or recommendations

   PT   Discharge examination and evaluation

Practice Exercise 5 ➤
Answers to numbers 2, 4, and 6 in Practice Exercise 5 are in the Instructor's Guide.

Answers to numbers 1, 3, and 5:
Mr. Jones
The pathology is fractured vertebra and severed spinal cord.
The impairment is paralyzed legs.
The functional limitation is the inability to stand or walk.
The disability is the inability to play football and return to his profession.

Mrs. Williams
The pathology is rheumatoid arthritis.
The impairment is limited ROM in knees and hips.
The functional limitation is the inability to climb stairs or steps.
The disability is the inability to live or function in an environment that contains stairs and steps.

Joe

The pathology is his head injury.

The impairment is his difficulty maintaining his balance and feeling dizzy.

The functional limitation is his inability to walk without the walker and without someone nearby.

The disability is his inability to take part in any walking activities that would require him to also use his hands, and he can never be alone when walking.

Practice Exercise 6 ➤   *Answers to Practice Exercise 6 are in the Instructor's Guide.*

CHAPTER 3   Practice exercises begin on page 44.

Practice Exercise 1 ➤   *Example:*

S: My car is saying "flap, flap, flap."

O: I feel the car pulling to the right. After stopping at the side of the road, I get out and observe that the right front tire is flat. After preparing the car to change the flat, I cannot turn the bolts. I observe rust around them.

A: Unable to meet goal to independently change flat tire. Need to seek help. Not able to go further in my car.

P: Will walk to nearest house to call AAA for help.

—Marianne Lukan

I want to drive the van to visit my daughter instead of making the trip in my little car. I went to the key rack to get the van keys and they were missing. Because my husband had been napping on the couch earlier in the day, I felt under the couch cushions. The keys to the van were there. The keys must have fallen out of his pocket when he was napping. I was able to take the van to visit my daughter. I will remind my husband to always hang the keys on the key rack instead of keeping them in his pocket.

—Marianne Lukan

Practice Exercise 2 ➤   **Dx:** Multiple sclerosis.

PT Dx: LE weakness limiting ability to sit ↔ stand and ambulate safely.

Patient expresses frustration—can't get up from couch without help, especially in evening.

Gross MMT 3 − /5 all LE muscle groups, 2/5 initial eval.

Observed patient sitting in middle of couch.

Patient sat at end of couch, scooted forward to edge, used couch arm to help push up.

3rd trial able to sit to stand Ⓘ Verbal cues to lean forward.

Instructed patient to not sit on couch in evening when fatigued and weaker.

Strength gain in LEs.

Goal Ⓘ sit to stand met.

Will visit patient 2 more times and schedule PT discharge evaluation.

Practice Exercise 3 ➤   3-26-00   **Dx:** Fx R femur, pinned 3-22-00.

PT Dx: Limited RLE mobility and NWB.

Pt. says he needs to be able to climb three flights of stairs to get to his apartment. Handrail on L going up. R ankle & foot edema. Circumference equals L foot & ankle measurements (see initial eval.). R knee flexion PROM 10–110°(15–100° last session). All R ankle AROM WNL. Pt. correctly demonstrated self knee ROM & gentle stretching exercises (see copy in chart).

Pt. ambulated, NWB R, axillary crutches, ①, on grass and uneven sidewalk, 300 ft. RLE mobility progressing. Pt. has met his short-term goal of independent crutch walking on level and uneven ground. Will work on stair climbing next session. Will inform PT that pt. will be ready for discharge evaluation next session.

—Confused Student, SPTA/Puzzled Therapist, PT (Lic. #420)

Practice Exercise 4 ➤   *Answers to Practice Exercise 4 are in the Instructor's Guide.*

Practice Exercise 5 ➤

DX: R CVA with L hemiplegia				INITIAL DATE: 2-24-00	
PRECAUTIONS: Broca's Aphasia, feeding tube				UPDATE: 3-25-00	

Exercise	Set	Rep	Equipment	Assist	Goals
Scapular protraction, supine L		5		Active assist	
L elbow extension, supine		5		tap muscle	1. Independent bed mobility
PROM/AAROM L UE & L LE	1	10		muscle belly	2. Independent unsupported sitting
PRE R UED1 & D2 diagonals, supine	1	10	2# cuff wt	tapping	3. Independent wheelchair mobility
	1	10	3# cuff wt	verbal cues	4. Standing pivot transfer with
	1	as many as he can, goal 10 reps 4#			minimum assist of 1
Resistive active exercise R LE					
SLR, abduction sidelying, prone	2	10	5# cuff wt	verbal cues	
knee flexion					
TKE long sitting	2	10	5# cuff wt		TDD:
					TDP:

Patient's Name	Age	Sex	MD	PT	RM#	Units
Harry A	71	M	Smith	Jones	E123	12

Transfers bed <-> w/c, w/c <-> mat table, w/c <-> toilet, w/c <-> straight chair	Method stand pivot to R side	Assist maximum x1	Other Practice squat pivot transfer w/c <-> mat moving towards L

Pregait/Gait

Amb x2 in //bars - max assist x2 - for wt shifting to L and knee control using temp AFO on L

Sitting balance in w/c with arms removed and in armless straight chair. Minimum assist x1. Work on head movement, eye tracking, wt shifting, trunk rot.

W/c mobility - room to bathroom, room to dining room, to PT department, to OT, speech. Check seating/cushion, L scapula protracted, arm on tray. Independent & brings self to department.

Practice Exercise 6 ➤

TOTAL KNEE ARTHROPLASTY

	Date 8-8-00		Date 8-9-00		Date 8-10-00		Date 8-11-00		Date 8-12-00	
CPM Degrees	am 25	pm 25	am 40	pm 40	am 60	pm 60	am 70	pm 70	am d/c by nursing	pm
CPM Time	1 hr on/1 hr off		same		same		same			
Knee ROM AA = Active Assist A = Active Supine			3 - 30	same	3 - 35	same	5 - 55	5 - 60	5 - 80	
Sitting			Pain, needs support		to 45	same	to 60	to 75	to 80	
Exercises: Isometrics Quads/Gluts/HS			Independent good coordination		Independent		same		I	
Ankle Pumps			Independent		Independent		same		I	
TKE					Independent		same		I	
SLR			Unable independent		Independent		min assist	Ind	I	
Active Knee Flex			Too painful to do		Independent		same		I	
Transfers: Bed Mobility			mod assist with leg		same		Independent		I	
Toilet/Commode									I	
Shower Seat									I	
Car Transfer									I	
Standing Pivot					yes		yes		yes	
Sliding Board										
Supine <--> Sit			mod assist knee supp		same		SBA		I	
Sit <--> Stand							Independent		I	
Balance: Sitting					good on edge of bed		same		I	
Standing			at side of bed		mod assist 1/walker				I	
Ambulation: Device			Too painful to start		walker		walker	crutches	crutches	
Weight Bearing			PWB R LE		PWB 50% body wt		PWB 75%		same	
Pattern									3 pt step thru	
Distance					few steps to chr/50'		50'x2	50'x1	125'	
Surface					level, tiled		tile,carpet	level	tile,carpet	
Assist					mod assist x1		SBA	min assist	Ind	
Stairs									SBA	
Blood Pressure					140/85 ā 145/88 p̄					
Pulse					72 bpm ā 100 bpm p̄					
Modalities	ice pack prn		continuous ice pack		same		d/c in am			
THERAPIST	Jennifer Nice, PT		Mary Jones, PTA		Mary Jones, PTA		Mary Jones, PTA		Mary Jones, PTA	

PHYSICAL THERAPY PROGRESS

PRECAUTIONS: Drain in place 8-8-00, 8-9-00 am, removed 8-9-00 pm

NAME: Earl

CHAPTER 4   Practice exercises begin on page 57.

Practice Exercise 1 ➤   9-17-00   **Dx:** Left total knee arthroplasty.

PT Dx: Dependent in ambulation, left lower extremity weakness, partial weight bearing allowed.

S: Patient states he slept "poorly" last two nights. Patient reported minimal complaints of pain with exercise during treatment session.

O: Patient transferred out of bed right supine to sit with moderate assist times one. Sat times five minutes with complaints of dizziness. Gait training with front wheeled walker partial weight bearing left flat surface times 30 feet moderate assist times one two times with 5-minute rest. Patient returned to bed for therapeutic exercise to left lower extremity of quadriceps set 10 repetitions 5 second hold with strong contraction. Straight leg raise times 10 repetitions with external rotation to decrease 10° lag. Active range of motion left knee 10–50°, passive range of motion 0–60°.

A: Increased range of motion, increased distance. Patient making gains even though not able to sleep well. Patient expected to achieve short-term goal of increased range of motion, increased strength, and minimum assist gait.

P: Continue gait training and therapeutic exercise. Begin stair ambulation afternoon 9/18/00.

—John Thomas, PTA lic#6411

Practice Exercise 2 ➤
1. No date and signature.
2. Many open spaces where someone could insert information or falsify the record.
3. Incorrect grammar and spelling.

Practice Exercise 3 ➤
1. Not full legal signature and no title.
2. Note not brief, some information not relevant to the problem of treatment.
3. Not clear (e.g., what does "lots of cheating" mean?).
4. Spelling and punctuation incorrect.
5. Error not initialed and dated.

Practice Exercise 4 ➤ *Answers to Practice Exercise 4 are in the Instructor's Guide.*

Practice Exercise 5 ➤ *Answers to Practice Exercise 5 are in the Instructor's Guide.*

CHAPTER 5 Practice exercises begin on page 70.

Practice Exercise 1 ➤

SD	Pt. states she has a clear understanding of her disease and her prognosis.
SD	Pt. expresses surprise that the ice massage relaxed her muscle spasm.
Pr	Muscle spasms L lumbar paraspinals with sitting tolerance limited to 10 min.
SD	Pt. describes tingling pain down back of R leg to heel.
Pr	Dependent in ADLs because of flaccid paralysis in R upper and lower extremities.
SD	Sue states her L ear hurts.
Pr	Unable to reach behind back because of limited ROM in R shoulder int. rot.
SD	Reports he must be able to return to work as a welder.
SD	Pt. states the doctor told her she had a laceration of R vastus medialis.
Pr	Paraplegic 2° SCI T_{12} and dependent in wheelchair transfers.
SD	States Hx of RA since 1980.
SD	Pt. denies pain $\bar{c}$ cough.
SD	States injury occurred December 31, 1999.
SD	SPTA c/o he has to sit for 2 hours in the PTA lectures.

    Pr   Grip strength weakness and inability to turn doorknobs to open doors because of carpal tunnel syndrome.

    SD   Describes his pain as "burning."

    Pr   Unable to sit because of decubitus over sacrum.

    Pr   Unable to feed self because of limited elbow flexion.

    SD   Pt. rates her pain a 4 on an ascending scale of 1–10.

    SD   States able to sit through a 2-hour movie last night.

Practice Exercise 2 ➤   1.   Pr   Muscle spasms L lumbar paraspinals with sitting tolerance limited to 10 min.

    Pr   Dependent in ADLs because of flaccid paralysis in R upper and lower extremities.

    Pr   Unable to reach behind back because of limited ROM in R shoulder int. rot.

    Pr   Paraplegic 2° SCI T_{12} and dependent in wheelchair transfers.

    Pr   Grip strength weakness and inability to turn doorknobs to open doors because of carpal tunnel syndrome.

    Pr   Unable to sit because of decubitus over sacrum.

    Pr   Unable to feed self because of limited elbow flexion.

    2.   SD   Pt. states she has a clear understanding of her disease and her prognosis.

    SD   Pt. expresses surprise that the ice massage relaxed her muscle spasm.

    SD   Pt. describes tingling pain down back of R leg to heel.

    SD   Sue states her L ear hurts.

    SD   Reports he must be able to return to work as a welder.

    SD   Pt. states her doctor told her she had a laceration of R vastus medialis.

    SD   States Hx of RA since 1980.

    SD   Pt. denies pain c̄ cough.

    SD   States injury occurred December 31, 1999.

    SD   SPTA c/o he has to sit for 2 hours in the PTA lectures.

    SD   Describes his pain as "burning."

    SD   Pt. rates her pain a 4 on an ascending scale of 1–10.

    SD   States able to sit through a 2-hour movie last night.

3. **Medical diagnoses:**
   Laceration
   SCI
   RA
   Carpal tunnel syndrome
   Decubitus

Practice Exercise 3 ➤

MISTAKES:

1. Used a pain scale, whereas the PT used a body drawing in the initial evaluation. One cannot compare a pain scale with a body drawing to document treatment effectiveness.

2. Talked about pain in the objective data section or did not write that the patient states or reports pain when lying propped on elbows or reports no pain in buttock area.

REWRITE:

6-3-00   **Dx:** Disc protrusion L4,5.

PT Dx: Muscle spasms lumbar paraspinals with limited sitting and sleeping tolerance, difficulty with ADLs, and unable to perform work tasks.

Pt. states she was able to sit through 30 minutes of "The Young and The Restless" soap opera yesterday. Marked body drawing with pain located in right low back, but not in buttock area. Colored markings green instead of red as in initial evaluation, indicating decreased pain intensity. See body drawing in chart. Before traction reported inability to tolerate lying propped on elbow because of pain in low back. Pt. has received 4 treatment sessions. Decrease in muscle tone palpable after 10 minute massage to right lumbar paraspinal muscles, prone position over one thin pillow. Able to lie propped on elbows 5 minutes following 10 minutes, prone, static pelvic traction, 70 lb. Correctly performed lumbar extension exercises 1, 2, and 3 of home exercise program (see copy in chart) and observed consistently using correct sitting posture with lumbar roll. Pt. required frequent verbal cueing for correct body mechanics while performing 10 reps (3 reps in initial eval.) of circuit of job simulation activities consisting of bed making, rolling and moving 30-lb (10-lb in initial eval.) dummy "patient" in bed, pivot transferring the dummy, and wheelchair handling. She did 10 back arches between each task without reminders. Pt. has reached 30-minute sitting tolerance goal, is independent with home exercise program and compliant with techniques for controlling the protrusion. Progress toward outcome of return to work is 60% with more consistent use of correct body mechanics and ability to lift 50-lb dummy required. Pt. to continue treatment sessions 33/week for 2 more weeks per PT's initial plan. Will notify PT that interim evaluation is scheduled for 6-7-00.

—Sue Smith, PTA, Lic. #0003

Practice Exercise 4 ➤   *Answers to the even numbered questions in Practice Exercise 4 are in the Instructor's Guide.*

____Yes____   1. Client stated her dog was hit by a car last night and she felt too depressed today to do her exercises.

____No____   3. Patient's daughter stated she traveled from Iowa, where it has been raining for 2 weeks.

____Yes____   5. Patient rates her pain a 4 on an ascending scale of 1–7.

____Yes____   7. Patient reports he had this same tingling discomfort in his right foot 3 years ago.

_____No_____ 9. Patient says she has 10 grandchildren and 4 great grandchildren.

_____No_____ 11. Client reports that "ER" is his favorite TV program.

_____Yes_____ 13. Client states he played golf yesterday for the first time since his back injury.

_____Yes_____ 15. Client states she cannot turn her head to look over her shoulder to back the car out of the garage.

_____No_____ 17. Client reports he wishes he had not been drinking beer the night of his accident.

_____No_____ 19. Client wishes it would rain as her prize roses are dying.

CHAPTER 6   Practice exercises begin on page 84.

Practice Exercise 1 ➤   *Answers to 3, 6, 9, 12, 15, and 18 in Practice Exercise 1 are in the Instructor's Guide.*

1. _____SD_____ Pt. c/o pain with prolonged sitting.

2. _____OD_____ Decubitus on sacrum measures 3 cm from L outer edge to R outer edge.

4. _____OD_____ R knee flexion PROM 30–90° .

5. _____OD_____ Ambulates c̄ standard walker, PWB L, bed to bathroom (20 ft), tiled surface, min assist 13 verbal cueing for gait pattern.

7. _____Pr_____ Limited ROM in L shoulder 2° to Fx greater tubercle of humerus and unable to put on winter coat without help.

8. _____SD_____ c/o itching in scar R knee.

10. _____Pr_____ Unable to feed self with L hand because of limited elbow ROM 2° Fx L olecranon process.

11. _____OD_____ AROM WNL bil. LEs.

13. _____Pr_____ Dependent in bed mobility because of dislocated R hip.

14. _____SD_____ Expresses concern over lack of progress.

16. _____SD_____ Kathy reports PTA courses are easy.

17. _____OD_____ Pt. pivot transfers, NWB R, bed ↔ w/c, max. assist of 2 for strength, balance, NWB cueing.

19. _____OD_____ LUE circumference at 3 cm superior to olecranon process is 12 cm.

20. _____OD_____ BP 125/80 mmHg, pulse 78 BPM, regular, strong.

Practice Exercise 2 ➤

1. 7. ___Pr___ Limited ROM in L shoulder 2° to Fx greater tubercle of humerus and (unable to put on winter coat without help.)

10. ___Pr___ (Unable to feed self with L hand) because of limited elbow ROM 2° Fx L olecranon process.

13. ___Pr___ (Dependent in bed mobility) because of dislocated R hip.

2. 1. ___SD___ Pt. c/o pain with prolonged sitting.

8. ___SD___ c/o itching in scar R knee.

14. ___SD___ Expresses concern over lack of progress.

16. ___SD___ Kathy reports PTA courses are easy.

3. 2. ___OD___ Decubitus on sacrum measures 3 cm from L outer edge to R outer edge.

4. ___OD___ R knee flexion PROM 30–90°

5. ___OD___ Ambulates c̄ standard walker, PWB L, bed to bathroom (20 ft), tiled surface, min. assist 1× for balance, verbal cueing for gait pattern.

11. ___OD___ AROM WNL bil. LEs.

17. ___OD___ Pt. pivot transfers, NWB R, bed ⟷ w/c, max assist of 2 for strength, balance, NWB cueing.

19. ___OD___ LUE circumference at 3 cm superior to olecranon process is 12 cm.

20. ___OD___ BP 125/80 mmHg, pulse 78 BPM, regular, strong.

4. **Medical diagnoses:**
Decubitus
Fx greater tubercle of humerus
Fx left olecranon process
Dislocated hip

Practice Exercise 3 ➤

1. Nothing wrong, documentation complete.

2. Measurement scale not consistent with initial exam. Used inches in progress note vs. centimeters in initial examination.

3. Right or left hip? Passive or active ROM? Which motion? The hip has six motions. No starting point for the measurement. What position was patient in?

4. Right or left? Measurement scale not the same as used in PT's initial examination.

5. No starting point for the measurement. It probably should read 0–20°.

6. Measurement sites not specific enough, no position of patient.

7. Blood pressure should be in mmHg, pulse in BPM, no position of patient, do not know when the measurements were taken (exercise or resting).

8. All measurements recorded in inches except for one, recorded in centimeters.

9. Nothing wrong, documentation complete.

10. The starting point of the measurements not documented. Active or passive motion?

11. Nothing wrong. Documentation complete.

12. Measurement landmarks not documented.

13. An estimate or judgment by observation. Not everyone will make the same judgment. Measurement technique not described.

14. No measurement technique described.

15. Nothing wrong. Documentation complete.

Practice Exercise 4 ➤

1. Cannot be reproduced. Need type of US, more specific target tissue, position of patient, time, purpose.

2. Cannot be reproduced. Need type of massage, patient position, purpose, more specific treatment area, time.

3. Can be reproduced. Documentation complete.

4. Cannot be reproduced. Need list or type of exercises, more specific as to treatment area (e.g., which motion?), patient position, repetitions.

5. Cannot be reproduced. Need type of traction equipment (static or intermittent), pounds, on/off time, duration, patient position, which muscles.

6. Cannot be reproduced. Need to know purpose.

7. Can be reproduced. Documentation complete. Assume all information is in written instructions in copy in chart.

8. Cannot be reproduced. Need dosage and time.

9. Cannot be reproduced. Need patient position, parameters or settings, electrode size, number, and placement, time or duration.

10. Can be reproduced. Documentation complete.

Practice Exercise 5 ➤

1. Following instructions, patient safely and independently ambulated no wt. bearing on right with axillary crutches 100 ft on tiled and carpeted level surfaces, was able to sit down and rise from bed, chair, toilet, and transfer in and out of car. She managed a flight of stairs with crutches and railing (on right going up) with verbal cueing. She safely managed two steps and curbs with crutches. Patient was provided with written crutch-walking instructions for reminders. See copy in chart.

2. Client performed circuit of brick layer job simulation activities for body mechanics training, 20 minutes, 15 repetitions for goal of returning to work. Client observed consistently using correct body mechanics and maintaining lumbar curve when lifting bricks and spreading mortar, but required verbal cueing to correct his tendency to bend and twist at the waist when wheeling and turning the wheelbarrow.

3. During transfer training, patient practiced sliding board transfers from wheelchair ⟷ toilet 3×, requiring frequent verbal cueing for safety precautions, and progressing from maximum assist to help push across the board to minimum assist on third transfer from chair to toilet. Moderate assist needed on third attempt to push from toilet back into chair.

4. During gait training patient ambulated with wide-based quad cane on left from bed to bathroom, to window, to hall in front of room, to wheelchair next to bed 5× with 2 minutes rest in chair between each circuit. He required minimum assist for wt. shifting to the right first 3 times, but demonstrated independent wt. shifting during the 4th and 5th walks. Patient independently recovered slight loss of balance 3×.

CHAPTER 7   Practice exercises begin on page 104.

Practice Exercise 1 ➤   **SITUATION A:**

Expected functional outcomes:

2. Patient will (able to manage) two steps with an assistive device and a railing and to manage car transfers for next visit to the doctor in 4 weeks.

Anticipated goals:

1. Pt. will consistently (move) up and down in bed and (roll) from side to side with SBA in 2 weeks.

2. Pt. will consistently (roll) to L side and (reach) for telephone and call bell with SBA in 3 weeks.

3. Pt. will consistently (move) from supine to sitting on edge of bed and (return) to supine position with minimal assist of 1 to help swing L leg into bed in 1 week.

4. Pt. will consistently (move) from sitting to standing and back to sitting from bed, toilet, wheelchair, standard chair with minimum assist of 1 for balance control and even weight bearing cueing in 2 weeks.

5. Using a quad cane, pt. will consistently (ambulate) bed to bathroom, and to meals with moderate assist of 1 for balance control and gait posture cueing in one week.

SITUATION B:

Expected functional outcomes: At anticipated discharge in 20 days, patient will (transfer) (and ambulate) independently for return to home.

1. Patient will independently and consistently (move) from sit to stand and stand to sit using elevated toilet seat, and all other surfaces no lower than 18 inches.

2. Patient will independently and consistently (walk) with a single-end cane on all surfaces and in the community.

Anticipated goals:

1. Pt. will consistently (be able to sit to stand and return) with standby assist (SBA) of 1 if boost is needed from edge of bed, elevated toilet seat, wheelchair, and standard dining room chair in 10 days.

2. Pt. will consistently be able to (ambulate) using a single-end cane for balance on tiled and carpeted level surfaces, to bathroom and dining room for meals with SBA of 1 for balance control in 10 days.

Practice Exercise 2 ➤
1. A. Increase right knee PROM to 0–90° in 1 week.
   B. In 1 week, pt. will be able to use 0–90° PROM in right knee to sit in narrow theater seat aisle for 30 minutes in preparation for return to work as a movie critic.

2. A. Sit unsupported and independently on edge of bed for 5 minutes in 3 days.
   B. In 3 days, pt. will be able to sit independently and without support on the edge of the bed for 5 minutes to eat her afternoon snack.

3. A. Ambulate 30 ft on tiled level surface, using standard walker, partial weight bearing on left, with standby assist for verbal cueing for gait pattern in 4 days.
   B. In 4 days, pt. will ambulate with standard walker for partial weight bearing on left, from bed to bathroom, with nursing assistant for standby assist for verbal cueing for safety.

4. A. Increase strength of left hip abductors from 3/5 to 4/5 in 3 weeks.
   B. In 3 weeks, patient's left hip abductors will have increased strength (4/5) to allow pt. to ambulate two city blocks without an assistive device and without a left trunk lean.

5. A. Decrease pain rating on pain scale from 6/10 to 3/10 in 4 treatment sessions.
   B. After 4 treatment sessions, pt. will rate pain 3/10 while demonstrating smooth movements and even weight bearing when performing nursing assistant job simulation tasks with proper body mechanics.

6. A. Will be able to safely perform job tasks so as to be able to return to work in 1 month.
   B. Patient will be able to lift and carry 50-lb boxes from conveyor belt to pallet and stack boxes on the pallet, using safe body mechanics and back protection techniques as required for his return to work in 1 month.

7. A. Patient will report decreased pain with movements in 1–2 weeks.
   B. Patient will demonstrate smooth movements when rising from bed, chair, and getting in and out of the car while reporting less pain in 1–2 weeks.

8. A. Edema in right thumb will be decreased to allow active ROM to be WNL in 3 weeks.
   B. Edema in right thumb will be decreased so patient will be able to use full ROM in the thumb to play his guitar.

9. A. Patient will report no pain when stepping down a 4-inch step in 4 weeks.
   B. In 4 weeks, patient will safely and smoothly descend the 4-inch steps required to reach the bottom of his steep embankment.

10. A. This is correctly written and is a functional outcome.

Practice Exercise 3 ➤   *Answers to Practice Exercise 3 are in the Instructor's Guide.*

Practice Exercise 4 ➤   4-17-00   **Dx:** R Colles' fracture, healed, cast removed.

PT Dx: Restricted ROM in wrist with inability to open doors, limited ability to grasp and pull for dressing activities.

S: Pt. reports able to put on panty hose today without help from husband and turned bathroom doorknob to open the door.

O: Pt. has been seen 23×. Pt. performed AROM exercises R forearm pronation/supination while in arm whirlpool, 110° F, 20 min to increase circulation and increase extensibility to R wrist tissues to prepare for stretching exercises. Contract–relax stretching techniques, 5 reps each, to increase pronation, supination and wrist extension ROM, sitting with forearm supported on table. Pt. correctly demonstrated home exercise program for strengthening finger flexion, wrist flexion and extension, forearm pronation and supination (see copy in chart). ROM today vs. 4-10-00:

	4-17-00	4-10-00
R pronation	0–50°	0–40°
R supination	0–70°	0–60°
Wrist extension	0–30°	0–20°

Grip strength 20 lb today, 10 lb 4-10-00. Pt. turned door handles and opened all inside doors in the clinic using R hand, but unable to turn handle and open door to outside. Able to grasp rope on scale and pull, exerting 3-lb force (2-lb 4-10-00).

A: Strengthening and stretching treatment procedures effective in increasing strength and ROM, improving progress toward goals of independent dressing activities and ability to open all types of doors.

P: To see pt. on 4-24-00 and notify PT discharge eval. to be 4-31-00. Will work on opening outside doors next visit.

—Sally Citizen, PTA, Lic. #5631

Practice Exercise 5 ➤   *Answers to Practice Exercise 5 are in the Instructor's Guide.*

Practice Exercise 6 ➤   1-20-00   **Dx:** Orthostatic hypotension 28 SCI C7

PT Dx: Unable to tolerate upright sitting.

S: Pt. continues to c/o dizziness when he attempts sitting.

O: Pt. has had 3 sessions on the tilt table to develop tolerance for upright sitting. First session BP dropped from 130/80 mmHg to 90/50 mmHg p̄ 10 min. at 40° elevation. Today BP dropped from 130/80 mmHg ā tx to 100/60 mm Hg p̄ 15 min. on tilt table at 50°. BP 125/75 mmHg 5 min p̄ pt. returned to supine position.

A: Progress toward outcome of upright sitting for 30 min is 50%. Severity of orthostatic hypotension is reduced. Blood pressure more stable with less drop than previous treatment sessions and with appropriate recovery.

Practice Exercise 7 ➤   11-2-00   **PT Dx:** Open wound due to 2nd-degree burn on L gluteus medius, not able to sit with even wt. bearing.

Pt. reports itching around edge of wound. Pt. sat in whirlpool 100° F, 20 min for wound debridement and to increase circulation for healing, sterile technique dressing change. No eschar, edges pink, 1 tsp. drainage, clear, odorless. Diameter R outer edge to L outer edge: 4 cm today compared to 4.8 cm 10-31-00. Pt. sat in whirlpool with even weight bearing on pelvis and taking support from arms on edge of whirlpool. Treatment is effective for goal to enhance wound healing process and closing for proper sitting. No evidence of infection.

Practice Exercise 8 ➤   *Write the interpretation of the data portion of this note:*

A: US effective in decreasing inflammation with a reduction in pain rating. Pt. on target for meeting anticipated goals. Goal #3 met for shoulder flexion and #2 for consistent use of proper body mechanics for lifting. Needs further training for proper reaching technique. Steady gains in ability to lift heavier objects to be able to load luggage in taxi trunk.

a. Are the subjective and objective data recorded correctly? Yes. Subjective information is relevant and pain rating is with the subjective data. Objective information is reproducible and patient's ability to do the functional tasks is described. Measurements are compared with previous measurements. Skilled physical therapy services are needed for body mechanics training and corrections.

b. Are the goals written correctly? Yes. Action verbs are reduced, use, increase; measurable criteria are pain rating, consistent proper body mechanics, range of motion measurements compared to initial exam results, up 50%; time period is 5 days for all three goals. All goals relate to the expected functional outcome.

Practice Exercise 9 ➤   *Write the interpretation of the data section of this note:*

A: ROM for rotation responding to stretching exercises by steadily gaining in degrees. On target for meeting goal #1. Independent in HEP except chin tucks; goal #2 95% met with monitoring of quality of chin tucks needed.

a. Are the subjective and objective data written properly? Yes. Subjective information is relevant. Objective information is reproducible. Measurements compared with previous results. Description of patient's quality of motion when doing the exercises is described. Skilled physical therapy services needed for training and corrections in the chin tuck exercise.

b. Are the goals written properly? Yes. Action verbs are *improve* and *performing;* measurable criteria are AROM, range of motion measurements, see objects at shoulder level, independent HEP; time periods are 2 weeks and 1 week. Goals relate to expected functional outcome.

Practice Exercise 10 ➤   *Answers to Practice Exercise 10 are in the Instructor's Guide.*

CHAPTER 8   Practice exercises begin on page 118.

Practice Exercise 1 ➤

1-20-00   **Dx:** Orthostatic hypotension 2° SCI C$_7$.

PT Dx: Unable to tolerate upright sitting.

S: Pt. continues to c/o dizziness when he attempts sitting.

O: Pt. has had 3 sessions on the tilt table to develop tolerance for upright sitting. First session BP dropped from 130/80 mmHg to 90/50 mmHg $\bar{p}$ 10 min at 40° elevation. Today BP dropped from 130/80 mmHg $\bar{a}$ tx to 100/60 mmHg $\bar{p}$ 15 min on tilt table at 50°. BP 125/75 mmHg 5 min $\bar{p}$ pt. returned to supine position.

A: Progress toward goal of upright sitting for 30 min is 50%. Severity of orthostatic hypotension decreasing. Blood pressure more stable with less drop than previous treatment sessions and with appropriate recovery.

P: Will continue tilt-table treatment bid per PT's plan until pt. tolerates 70° for 20 min then consult PT about when to try sitting in chair with back that reclines.

—Kathy A. Student, SPTA/Marianne Lukan, PT Lic. #xxx

Practice Exercise 2 ➤

11-2-00   **PT Dx:** Open wound due to 2nd-degree burn on L gluteus medius, not able to sit with even wt. bearing.

Pt. reports itching around edge of wound. Pt. sat in whirlpool 100°, 20 min for wound debridement and to increase circulation for healing, sterile technique dressing change. No eschar, edges pink, 1 tsp. drainage, clear, odorless. Diameter R outer edge to L outer edge: 4 cm today compared to 4^3/$_4$ cm 10-31-85. Treatment is effective for goal to enhance wound healing process and closing for proper sitting. No evidence of infection. Will continue treatment daily per PT's plan until open area measures 2 cm and consult PT about time to begin ambulation.

—Jerry A. Student, SPTA/Marianne Lukan, PT Lic. #xxx

Practice Exercise 3 ➤

INTERVENTION PLAN #1:

2. (Exercises), including home program, for hip abductor muscles to strengthen to grade 5/5.

3. Home program of structured, progressive (walking and stair climbing) activities to increase tolerance to the activities without aggravating the bursitis.

Frequencies: 3×/week and 2×/week ; Duration: total 4 weeks

INTERVENTION PLAN #2:

1. (Exercises) to strengthen all extremities to aid transfers and ambulation. Exercise plan to include home program.

2. (Training and practice for transfers) from all types of surfaces as required in the home.

3. (Gait training) with platform walker on level tiled and carpeted surfaces and one step as required in the home.

4. (Home assessment visit) to clarify needs for transfer and gait training planning.

5. (Educate) patient and family on hip protection and safety precautions for safe functioning in the home.

Frequency: twice daily (bid); duration: 2 weeks.

INTERVENTION PLAN #3:

1. Home program of (exercises) to increase ROM and strength of L elbow and hip in preparation for ambulation with cane and independent ADLs.

2. (Transfer and ambulation training) with progression of assistive devices appropriate for safe change from platform walker to goal of single-end cane.
3. (Ambulation training) on grass and dock using assistive device.
4. (Stair climbing training) with assistive device and railing in home and into motor home.

Frequencies: 3×/week and then 2×/week; duration: 2 weeks then 1 week for a total of 3 weeks.

CHAPTER 9   Practice exercises begin on page 128.

Practice Exercise 1 ➤   **Name:** Janet Smith   **Room #:** 102   **MR #:** 2001   **Date:** 11/15/00

Pt. has orders for PT daily for strengthening exercises, transfer training, and gait training with walker. She declined treatment today, stating her RLE was "too sore and swollen from being up in wheelchair too long." Writer notes T.E.D.s socks on RLE with minimal edema at lateral malleolus, LEs elevated in bed at this time. Nurse's note reflects pt.'s request for increased Tylenol, which is medication provided pt. as needed. Encouraged pt. to perform isometric LE exercises previously instructed on while in bed. Plan to see for treatment tomorrow.

—Diane Palmstein, PTA/Mary Smith, PT

Practice Exercise 2 ➤

```
                    ABC HEALTH CENTER
                     INCIDENT REPORT
```

Resident/Visitor #1: Mr. X	Resident/Visitor #2: NA
Address: Room 201	Address:
Phone #: DOB 07/08/20	Phone #: DOB_____
Date: 12/01/00 Time 10:20 (am)/pm	Location of Incident: Room 201

Description of Incident: Pt. is transfering from wheelchair to bed with a walker and with PTA on ℝ side, holding transfer belt. During pivot, pt's ℝ knee buckles. PTA guides pt down onto the bed but the bed rolls back. PTA lowers pt to floor and rests pt's head and back against the PTA. Pt is in a semi reclined position with both legs straight out in front. PTA calls for help.

Assessment: Describe injury (if any) in detail:

Pt c̄ pain in ℝ buttocks, denies pain in ℝ hip or leg. No injury identified by physician.

Name/Title of All Witnesses:	Safety Measures in Use:
Marianne Lukas PTA	Transfer Belt: X Siderails:_____ Restraint:_____ Type:_____

Intervention: None Required _____   At Facility X

Describe: Jane Doe RN and Tom Jones, NA, assisted PTA in lifting Mr. X from floor to bed. Dr. Young examined pt. No injury identified, but pt may have bumped buttocks on bed siderail. Pt to remain in bed and RN will monitor skin condition and pain complaints for remainder of the day.

Resident #1 Mr. X

Hospitalized: Yes___ No X	Date NA Time____am/pm	Hospital NA
Physician Name: Dr. Young	Notified by: Jane Doe RN Date 12-1-00 Time 10:30 (am)/pm	
Family Name: Mrs. X	Notified by: Jane Doe, RN Date 12-1-00 Time 11:00 (am)/pm	

Resident #2 NA

Hospitalized: Yes___ No___	Date_____ Time____am/pm	Hospital_____
Physician Name:	Notified by: Date_____Time____am/pm	
Family Name:	Notified by: Date_____Time____am/pm	

PREDISPOSING CONDITIONS

Diagnosis: Fx ℞ hip, repaired with prosthesis

Mental Status (i.e., Oriented, Alert/Confused, etc.): — Alert oriented

List pertinent medications if applicable:
Tylenol prn

Follow-Up Measures to Incident:
monitor ℞ buttock pain complaints. Resume PT. 12-2-00

Was a Medical Device Involved?   ☐ Yes   ☒ No   **Manufacturer's Name and Address (If Available on Equipment or Packaging):**

Type_____   Model No. _____

Serial No. _____   Lot No. _____

Incident Reported By: marianne Lukas   **Title:** PTA

Date of Report: 12-1-00	Signature & Title of Person Preparing Report: marianne Lukas PTA

Reviewed by DON:_____
(Signature)

Date:_____ Charted: ☐ Yes ☐ No

Reviewed by Administrator:_____
(Signature)

Date:_____

Reviewed by Medical Director:_____ **Date:**_____
(Signature or Initials)

DO NOT WRITE BELOW THIS LINE TO BE COMPLETED BY ADMINISTRATOR/DON

Vulnerable Adult Report Made?   Yes ☐   No ☐

Incident Reported To (Circle as many of the following as applicable.):

Local Welfare Agency   Local Police Department   County Sheriff's Office   Office of Health Facility Complaints

Other (Explain)_____

Date Report Called In (Within 5 Days):_____   **Approximate Time:**_____ ☐ a.m. ☐ p.m.

Name of Person Spoken to:_____   **Reported By:**_____

Date Report Mailed:_____   **To Whom:**_____

Safety lesson: Always lock brakes on wheeled beds

CHAPTER 10   Practice exercises begin on page 143.

Practice Exercise 1 ➤   **PROGRESS NOTE 1:**

PT Dx: Pt. has a decubitus over L lat. malleolus interfering with ability to wear proper shoe for ambulation.

S: She states, "It is Christmas and I don't have my shopping done."

O: Observed pt. scratching at her wound dressings. Wound dressing half off upon arrival to dept. Wound measures 3 cm horizontally across outer edge to outer edge (4 cm initial eval.), loose necrotic tissue, no drainage. Foot whirlpool 104°F, loose tissue dislodged, and dressings changed.

A: 50% progress toward goal of clean, healing wound to prepare for ambulation.

P: Will consult PT re: designing wrap over bandage to keep pt. from pulling dressing loose.

PROGRESS NOTE 2:

PT Dx: Pt is 82 YO c̄ terminal CA.

Subjective data: Pt. states he wants to go home. Pt.'s wife says she cannot care for pt. at home.

Objective data: Gluteus maximus and quads 3/5. Major mm groups in LEs 3/5 to 4/5 strength range. Pt. demonstrated 3 reps each of LE strengthening exercises to be performed in the ward with wife's help (see copy in chart). Maximum assist for transfer bed ⟷ commode ⟷ w/c. He needs max. assistance for sit ⟷ stand for strength to get up and for control when sitting down. Pt. ambulated 3× the length of the // bars (about 30 ft) c̄ min. assist for sense of security with verbal cues for posture and heel–toe stepping.

Interpretation of the data: Pt. is not independent in ADLs because of muscle weaknesses.

Plan: Will continue to work to ↑ mm strength and try sliding board transfers this PM.

Practice Exercise 2 ➤ *Answers to Practice Exercise 2 are in the Instructor's Guide.*

Practice Exercise 3 ➤   **3-26-00**   **PT Dx:** R foot edema.

Pt. says he needs to be able to climb three flights of stairs to get to his apartment. Handrail on L going up. Circumference equal L foot measurements. R knee flexion 10–110°. Pt. crutch walked NWB, 300 ft on grass outside c̄ no assistance. Pt. showing good progress in LE mobility. Pt. has met his short-term goal of independent crutch walking. Will work on stair climbing next session.

—Jim Jones, PTA

Note could be better written if:

PT Dx had a functional limitation.
PT Dx related to the treatment.
Legal guidelines were followed.

Subjective data: correct.

Objective data: if the measurement landmarks and position of patient were documented so measurements of circumference could be duplicated; if the position of patient for ROM measurements were described; if we knew whether measurements are consistent with initial examination, and if ROM measurements were compared with previous measurements; if ambulation description told the reader the type of crutches or how the pt.'s posture looked.

Interpretation of the data: if there was evidence to support the conclusion that LE mobility has improved; if the note recorded any treatment for the edema or the ROM problem, to support the documentation of the measurements; if it told how the measurements relate to crutch walking; if it talked about where pt. is independent crutch walker (in hospital? in community? in home?); if it described the functional outcome.

Plan: if PT involvement is mentioned; if the reader is told when pt. will be discharged; if it recorded how many more treatment sessions; if the note described a quality or thorough treatment session.

Practice Exercise 4 ➤   **PROGRESS NOTE 1:**

This is a poor note. It does not follow any of the guidelines for quality documentation. It talks about what the therapist did, in vague terms, and does not relate to the problems or how the patient is progressing. Information is organized properly and legal guidelines have been followed.

PROGRESS NOTE 2:

Large space at end of S section that needs a line drawn through. Better description of treatment, but treatment cannot be duplicated accurately. Target tissue for US not identified, position of patient, type of application (direct contact or immersion). Discussion of stretching exercises does not indicate patient's position or repetitions. We do not know whether the ROM was active or passive. We do not know how far pt. ambulated, quality of gait and posture, type of surfaces. We really don't know whether US and exercise increased ankle ROM. Maybe only the US helped, or maybe only the exercise helped. Goal of independent ambulation doesn't tell reader where or how far the ambulation is required. Cannot measure this goal. Plan does not state frequency or duration or thoughts as to what will happen next session to progress the pt. It is good to see a PT involved.

PROGRESS NOTE 3:

US treatment description much better. Position of pt. not mentioned, but reader could assume that the pt. was sitting because it was immersion US. Pain rating belongs in the subjective section. Stretching exercises still cannot be duplicated because we do not know patient's position or number of repetitions pt. tolerated. Nice visual for comparison of ROM measurements. We do not know what position was used when measurements were taken. We still do not know if it is AROM or PROM. A better description of the exercise program and purpose. Can visualize the patient ambulating and understand the relationship between the ankle problem and the gait. Which is more effective, US or exercise or both? What is planned for next session? How many more sessions will the pt. receive?

PROGRESS NOTE 4:

Excellent note. Needs some punctuation in the first sentence. Reader can duplicate US treatment and even know which machine to use (1 MHz). Demonstration of US effectiveness. We still do not know patient's positioning for stretching exercises, but can now assume patient was sitting. We continue not to know whether ROM measurements were taken with patient sitting or in another position and whether it was active or passive ROM. An insurance representative can see that the treatment is effective in progressing the patient toward independent functioning and taking responsibility for his or her own exercises. The reader is also told that the treatments will not go on for long, but an anticipated discharge date is soon.

Practice Exercise 5 ➤   Legal guidelines followed. Subjective data appropriate. Able to reproduce stretching exercises and knee measurements. Measurements compared with previous ones. Able to visualize the patient ambulating. Observed the independent use of walker in the patient's environment to confirm the subjective information. Treatment relates to the problems; transfers/ambulation and knee stretching were described. Assessment section relates relevance of increased knee flexion to function and measures progress toward goals. Plan does not tell reader frequency or duration of remaining treatment sessions.

Practice Exercise 6 ➤   (Note from Chapter 4, Practice Exercise 3)

11-17-00   **Dx:** L CVA.

PT Dx: R hemiparesis interfering with safe transfers, ambulation, and independent ADLs.

Pt. admits she has not been doing her home exercise program. Does not feel like going out to church or her club meetings because she is afraid of falling. Pt. practiced transferring from floor to chair 3× with minimum assistance to help push up from kneeling position to chair seat to enable her to get up if she were to fall. Pt. required frequent verbal cueing for sequencing the movements required to roll and sit up; demonstrated inability to bear wt. on R hand because of mild flexion contractures in all finger joints, and was able to independently move from supine to sit by rolling to R side, use R elbow for support, and push up to sitting with LUE. ~~PROM~~ AAROM exercises/supine on floor/for all RUE motions/10 reps each/ requiring minimal physical assistance but many verbal cues. Pt. demonstrated isometric shoulder exercises sitting, but required many reminders not to lean trunk. Pt. has difficulty remembering transfer and exercise instructions. Making slow progress toward goal of safe transfers. Treatment to continue 3× /week for 1 week and will schedule interim evaluation with PT for 11-24-00.

—Marianne Lukan, PTA Lic#2719

Practice Exercise 7 ➤ 7.1.

7-17-00   **PT Dx:** Decreased ROM & strength RLE limiting ambulation, Ⓘtransfers and bed mobility.

Pt. stated he was able to sit on a high stool in the tub, swing his leg over and then stand to take a shower today with wife standing by to help swing his leg. He denied pain today, but reported experiencing intense muscle spasms after sitting in his easy chair, also feeling a "clink" in hip area with his extension exercise. Pt. ambulated through all rooms on first floor with one crutch on L, demonstrating good balance, erect posture, 3-point step-through gait, with supervision for verbal cues for heel–toe gait.Ⓘstairs in home and porch, using one crutch and railing. Correctly performed 10 reps each exercises: standing at kitchen counter—toe raises, partial knee bends, hip abd., gentle hyperextension, hamstring curls; supine—SLR with approx 60–70% assist, bent knee abd.; sitting—long arc quads. Recommended he stop the hyperextension exercise if he feels " clink" again. Suggested they have easy chair raised by putting on platform and use 2 crutches when fatigued. Pt. smiling and pleasant, no longer presents with flat affect. Goal #3 met, but exercises ready to be progressed and pt. needs powder board for hip abduction. Progressing quickly toward goals 1 and 2, may be able to go to a cane, continues to need assist lifting R leg when transferring. Will bring powder board next visit on 7-25-00, monitor exercise program, and continue toward goals in PT's initial eval.

—Joe Jones, PTA Lic#007

7.2. *Draw lines through long spaces at end of sentences.*

Good that subjective statement is in quotation marks.

Pain complaint should go in subjective section. Better to have pt. rate the pain on a scale.

Note is about what the PTA did, not how the pt. performed. Cannot picture the patient and cannot duplicate the treatment. Need to describe how pt. looks when ambulating, how much assistance needed and why, how far or for how long ambulating, type of surfaces, assistance required on stairs. Need to describe the exercises or refer to copy in chart. Statement about pt. telling PTA how much wt. he is bearing belongs in subjective section. (PTA should measure or determine how much wt. pt. is bearing.)

No evidence in the S or O sections to support the A comments. How did PTA determine the progress was 90%? Why does pt. need 2 more visits?

7.3. This note follows all the guidelines.

7.4. a. Impairments: decreased strength, ROM, endurance

Functional limitations: transfers, bed mobility, sit ⟷ stand, ambulation.

b. (1) Safe andⒾ (transfers) from variety of surfaces in home ~~in 3 weeks~~.

(2) Safe andⒾhousehold (ambulation) with appropriate ambulation device for 5 or more minutes, up/down stairs to exit home ~~in 3 weeks~~.

(3) Wife/pt. to (carry out home exercise program) correctly andⒾ

   c. (1) Home program of ROM and strengthening (exercises) to increase ROM and strength of RLE to allow safe and Ⓘ transfers.
      (2) (Structured home ambulation program) to increase ambulation endurance to 5 min and to improve safety.
      (3) (Gait training) on stairs to allow exit from home.
      (4) (Transfer training) from a variety of surfaces with emphasis on getting in/out of bed.

   Treatment will be 2×/week ~~for 3 weeks~~.

   Impairments will be treated by exercises to increase strength & ROM and structured, progressive ambulation to increase endurance.

   Functional activities are transfers from variety of surfaces, ambulation, and stair climbing.

Practice Exercise 8 ➤

8.1. There are no subjective data because the PT did not write what the pt. said or told her or him. Because pt. was confused, the subjective data would not be relevant.

8.2. Yes, the objective data paint a picture of the wounds by describing how they look and giving measurements.

8.3. Yes, the data are reproducible. Another PT could describe the same appearances and perform the same measurements, although measurement on R does not describe the boundaries of the measurements.

8.4. Impairments are the pressure ulcers/open wounds with necrotic tissue and blister.

8.5. Functional limitations are dependent bed mobility and transfers.

8.6. Purpose of the treatment is to clean the wound of necrotic tissue and loose skin, enhance healing. Pt. should be able to improve in bed mobility and to perform assisted standing transfers when heels are healed.

8.7. Frequency 1×/day, and duration = 3 days.

8.8. (Debride) necrotic tissue ~~in 3 days~~ for clean wound with healthy tissue to enhance healing for eventual assisted bed mobility and assisted pivot transfers.

8.9. Yes, I can duplicate the treatment if I follow standard Pulsavac procedure. I know to do the treatment at bedside, and where to position towels. I also know sterile technique was used, since I am told the towels were sterile.

   There are only 3 treatments planned, so I will have the PT do the discharge eval. on the third treatment.

   I can document progress by describing how the wounds look and compare that description with the initial examination. I can measure and compare the measurements, and I can put the descriptions and measurements in chart form with initial examination data listed for comparison.

Practice Exercise 9 ➤

9.1. Documentation is evidence that may be needed years later.

9.2. Documentation is a legal record.

9.3. Medicare influenced history of documentation.

9.4. Legal guidelines.

9.5. Topic of impairment, functional limitation, and disability introduced.

9.6. Poor documentation raises questions and makes it difficult to recall information

9.7. How good documentation should look. A peek at what the book is about and how the student will be expected to document.

9.8. Abbreviations.

9.9. SOAP format.

9.10. Recording of license number.

9.11. Introduction to history of documentation.

9.12. Standards and criteria mentioned.

➤ APPENDIX F

Guidelines for Physical Therapy Documentation*

PREAMBLE The American Physical Therapy Association (APTA) is committed to meeting the physical therapy needs of society, to meeting the needs and interests of its members, and to developing and improving the art and science of physical therapy, including practice, education, and research. To help meet these responsibilities, the APTA Board of Directors has approved the following guidelines for physical therapy documentation. It is recognized that these guidelines do not reflect all of the unique documentation requirements associated with the many specialty areas within the physical therapy profession. Applicable for both handwritten and electronic documention systems, these guidelines are intended to be used as a foundation for the development of more specific documentation guidelines in specialty areas, while at the same time providing guidance for the physical therapy profession across all practice settings.

OPERATIONAL DEFINITIONS *Guidelines:* APTA defines "guidelines" as approved, nonbinding statements of advice.
Documentation: Any entry into the client record, such as: consultation report, initial examination report, progress note, flowsheet/checklist that identifies the care/service provided, reexamination report, or summation of care.
Authentication: The process used to verify that an entry is complete, accurate, and final. Indications of authentication can include original written signatures and computer "signatures" on secured electronic record systems only.

I. General Guidelines
A. All documentation must comply with the applicable jurisdictional/regulatory requirements.
   1. All handwritten entries should be made in ink and will include original signatures. Electronic entries should be made with appropriate security and confidentiality provisions.
   2. Informed consent: as required by the *APTA Standards of Practice for Physical Therapy and the Criteria.*
      2.1 The physical therapist has sole responsibility for providing information to the patient and for obtaining the patient's informed consent in accordance with jurisdictional law before initiating physical therapy.
      2.2 Those deemed competent to give consent are competent adults. When the adult is not competent, and in the case of minors, a parent or legal guardian consents as the surrogate decision maker.
      2.3 The information provided to the patient should include the following: (a) a clear description of the treatment ordered or recommended, (b) material (decisional) risks associated with the proposed treatment, (c) expected benefits

*Adopted by the Board of Directors
March, 1997.
Amended March 1993, June 1993, November 1994, March 1995, March 1997, November 1998.
From American Physical Therapy Association: *Guidelines for Physical Therapy Documentation. Guide to Physical Therapist Practice.* Alexandria, VA, July 1999, pp Appendix 7-1 to 7-3, with permission of the APTA.

of treatment, (d) comparison of the benefits and risks possible with and without treatment, and (e) reasonable alternatives to the recommended treatment. The physical therapist should solicit questions from the patient and provide answers. The patient should be asked to acknowledge understanding and consent before treatment proceeds.

Examples of ways in which to accomplish this documentation:

2.3.1 Signature of patient/guardian on long or short consent form,

2.3.2 Notation/entry of what was explained by the physical therapist or the physical therapist assistant in the official record, and

2.3.3 Filing of a completed consent checklist signed by the patient.

3. Charting errors should be corrected by drawing a single line through the error and initialing and dating the chart or through the appropriate mechanism for electronic documentation that clearly indicates that a change was made without deletion or the original record.

4. Identification.

   4.1 Include patient's full name and identification number, if applicable, on all official documents.

   4.2 All entries must be dated and authenticated with the provider's full name and appropriate designation (eg, PT, PTA).

   4.3 Documentation by students (SPT/SPTA) shall be authenticated by a licensed physical therapist.

   4.4 Documentation by graduates (GPT/GPTA) or others pending receipt of an unrestricted license shall be authenticated by a licensed physical therapist.

5. Documentation should include the referral mechanism by which physical therapy services are initiated.

   Examples include:

   5.1 Self-referral/direct access.

   5.2 Request for consultation from a practitioner.

   5.3 File copy of correspondence to referral source as acknowledgement of the referral.

II. Initial Examination and Evaluation/Consultation

A. Documentation is required at the onset of each episode of physical therapy care.

B. Elements include:

1. Obtaining a history and identifying risk factors.

   1.1 History of the presenting problem, current complaints, and precautions (including onset date).

   1.2 Pertinent diagnoses and medical history.

   1.3 Demographic characteristics, including pertinent psychological, social, and environmental factors.

   1.4 Prior or concurrent services related to the current episode of physical therapy care.

   1.5 Comorbidities that may affect goals and treatment plan.

   1.6 Statement of patient's knowledge of problem.

   1.7 Goals of patient (and family members and significant others, if appropriate).

2. Selecting and administering tests and measures to determine patient status in a number of areas.

   The following is a partial list of these areas, with illustrative tests and measures:

   2.1 Arousal, mentation, and cognition.

       Examples include objective findings related, but not limited, to the following areas:

       2.1.1 Level of consciousness.

       2.1.2 Ability to process commands.

       2.1.3 Alertness.

       2.1.4 Gross expressive and receptive language deficits.

    2.2 Neuromotor development and sensory integration.
Examples include objective findings related, but not limited, to the following areas:
        2.2.1 Gross and fine motor skills
        2.2.2 Reflex and movement patterns
        2.2.3 Dexterity, agility, and coordination
    2.3 Range of motion.
Examples include objective findings related, but not limited, to the following areas:
        2.3.1 Extent of joint motion
        2.3.2 Pain and soreness of surrounding soft tissue
        2.3.3 Muscle length and flexibility
    2.4 Muscle performance.
Examples include objective findings related, but not limited, to the following areas:
        2.4.1 Strength
        2.4.2 Power
        2.4.3 Endurance
    2.5 Ventilation, respiration, and circulation.
Examples include objective findings related, but not limited, to the following areas:
        2.5.1 Vital signs
        2.5.2 Breathing patterns
        2.5.3 Heart sounds
    2.6 Posture.
Examples include objective findings related, but not limited, to the following areas:
        2.6.1 Static posture
        2.6.2 Dynamic posture
    2.7 Gait, locomotion, and balance.
Examples include objective findings related, but not limited, to the following areas:
        2.7.1 Characteristics of gait
        2.7.2 Functional ambulation
        2.7.3 Characteristics of balance
    2.8 Self-care and home management status.
Examples include objective findings related, but not limited, to the following areas:
        2.8.1 Activities of daily living
        2.8.2 Functional capacity
        2.8.3 Static and dynamic strength
    2.9 Community and work (job/school/play) integration/reintegration.
Examples include objective findings related, but not limited, to the following areas:
        2.9.1 Instrumental activities of daily living
        2.9.2 Functional capacity
        2.9.3 Adaptive skills

3. Evaluation (a dynamic process in which the physical therapist makes clinical judgments based on data gathered during the examination).

4. Diagnosis (a label encompassing a cluster of signs and symptoms, syndromes, or categories that reflects the information obtained from the examination).

5. Goals.
    5.1 Patient (and family members or significant others, if appropriate) is involved in establishing goals.
    5.2 All goals are stated in measurable terms.

          5.3   Goals are linked to impairments, functional limitations, and disabilities identified in the examination.

          5.4   Short- and long-term goals are established when applicable. (May include potential for achieving goals.)

     6. Intervention plan or recommendation requirements:

          6.1   Shall be related to realistic goals and expected functional outcomes.

          6.2   Should include frequency and duration to achieve the stated goals.

          6.3   Should include patient and family/caregiver educational goals.

          6.4   Should involve appropriate collaboration and coordination of care with other professionals/services.

     7. Authentication and appropriate designation of physical therapist.

III. Documentation of the Continuum of Care

A. Intervention or service provided.

    1. Documentation is required for each patient visit/encounter. Authentication is required for every note by the physical therapist or the physical therapist assistant providing the service under the supervision of the physical therapist.
Examples include:

       1.1   Checklist

       1.2   Flow sheet

       1.3   Graph

       1.4   Narrative

    2. Elements may include:

       2.1   Identification of specific interventions provided.

       2.2   Equipment provided.

B. Patient status, progress, or regression

    1. Documentation is required for every visit/encounter. Authentication is required for every note by the physical therapist or the physical therapist assistant providing the service under the supervision of the physical therapist.

    2. Elements may include:

       2.1   Subjective status of patient.

       2.2   Changes in objective and measurable findings as they relate to existing goals.

       2.3   Adverse reaction to treatment.

       2.4   Progression/regression of existing therapeutic regimen, including patient education and compliance.

       2.5   Communication/consultation with providers/patient/family/significant other.

       2.6   Authentication and appropriate designation of either a physical therapist or a physical therapist assistant.

C. Reexamination and reevaluation.

    1. Documentation is required monthly for patients seen at intervals of a month or less; if the patient is seen less frequently, documentation is required for every visit or encounter.

    2. Elements include:

       2.1   Documentation of elements as identified in III.B.2.1 through III.B.2.5 to update patient's status.

       2.2   Interpretation of findings and, when indicated, revision of goals.

       2.3   When indicated, revision of treatment plan, as directly correlated with documented goals.

       2.4   Authentication and appropriate designation of physical therapist.

IV. Summation of Care

A. Documentation is required following conclusion of the current episode in the physical therapy care sequence.

B. Elements include:

    1. Reason for discontinuation of service.

Examples include:

1.1 Satisfactory goal achievement.

1.2 Patient declines to continue care.

1.3 Patient is unable to continue to work toward goals due to medical or psychosocial complications.

2. Current physical/functional status.

3. Degree of goal achievement and reasons for goals not being achieved.

4. Discharge plan that includes written and verbal communication related to the patient's continuing care.

Examples include:

4.1 Home program.

4.2 Referrals for additional services.

4.3 Recommendations for follow-up physical therapy care.

4.4 Family and caregiver training.

4.5 Equipment provided.

5. Authentication and appropriate designation of physical therapist.

REFERENCES   *Direction, Delegation and Supervision in Physical Therapy Services.* HOD 06-96-30-4.

Comprehensive Accreditation Manual for Hospitals. Oakbrook Terrace, Ill: Joint Commission on Accreditation of Healthcare Organizations; 1996.

Glossary of Terms Related to Information Security. Schaumburg, Ill: Computer-Based Patient Record Institute; 1996.

Guidelines for Establishing Information Security Policies at Organizations Using Computer-Based Patient Records. Schamburg, Ill: Computer-Based Patient Record Institute; 1995.

➤ INDEX

Page numbers followed a "b" indicate a box; page numbers followed by an "f" indicate a figure; page numbers followed by a "t" indicate a table.